Review Manual for

Massachusetts General Hospital Handbook of General Hospital Psychiatry

Review Manual for

Massachusetts General Hospital Handbook of General Hospital Psychiatry

Fifth Edition

Theodore A. Stern, MD, FAPM
Professor of Psychiatry,
Harvard Medical School;
Psychiatrist and Chief,
Psychiatric Consultation Service,
Massachusetts General Hospital,
Boston, Massachusetts

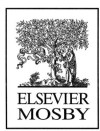

ELSEVIER
MOSBY

ELSEVIER
MOSBY

The Curtis Center
170 S Independence Mall W 300E
Philadelphia, Pennsylvania 19106

REVIEW MANUAL FOR MASSACHUSETTS GENERAL HOSPITAL
HANDBOOK OF GENERAL HOSPITAL PSYCHIATRY   ISBN 0-323-02768-7

Notice

Medicine is an ever-changing field. Standard safety precautions must be followed, but as new research and clinical experience broaden our knowledge, changes in treatment and drug therapy may become necessary or appropriate. Readers are advised to check the most current product information provided by the manufacturer of each drug to be administered to verify the recommended dose, the method and duration of administration, and contraindications. It is the responsibility of the treating physician, relying on experience and knowledge of the patient, to determine dosages and the best treatment for each individual patient. Neither the Publisher nor the author assume any liability for any injury and/or damage to persons or property arising from this publication.

The Publisher

Library of Congress Cataloging-in-Publication Data

Review manual for Massachusetts General Hospital handbook of general hospital psychiatry, fifth edition / [edited by] Theodore A. Stern.
    p.; cm.
    ISBN 0-323-02768-7
    1. Psychiatric consultation–Handbooks, manuals, etc. 2. Hospital patients–Mental health–Handbooks, manuals, etc. 3. Sick–Psychology–Handbooks, manuals, etc. I. Stern, Theodore A. II. Massachusetts General Hospital handbook of general hospital psychiatry.
    [DNLM: 1. Mental Disorders–Problems and Exercises. 2. Hospitalization–Problems and Exercises. 3. Patients–psychology–Problems and Exercises. 4. Psychology, Medical–Problems and Exercises. 5. Referral and Consultation–Problems and Exercises.
WM 18.2 R454 2004]
RC455.2.C65R485 2004
616'.001' 9–dc22

                                                                    2004052412

Printed in the United States of America

Last digit is the print number: 9 8 7 6 5 4 3 2 1

Preface

Never has the future of psychosomatic medicine looked brighter than it does now. The Academy of Psychosomatic Medicine (APM) is thriving, and the theme of the 2005 Annual Meeting of the American Psychiatric Association in Atlanta, Georgia is psychosomatic medicine. Moreover, psychosomatic medicine is now a newly-approved subspecialty; the first board examinations will be given June 4–7, 2005. For those interested in reviewing the field (either for a clinical update or to facilitate passage of the first subspecialty examination in Psychosomatic Medicine), several textbooks, including the recently published *Massachusetts General Hospital Handbook of General Hospital Psychiatry*, fifth edition (Mosby/Elsevier), summarize existing knowledge and practice patterns, as well as present new findings. In addition, board preparation courses (organized by the Massachusetts General Hospital's Department of Psychiatry and by the Academy of Psychosomatic Medicine) have been and will be offered.

Enthusiasm for the field is growing; practitioners who work at the interface of psychiatry and medicine are striving to solidify their knowledge and to break new ground. This volume of 800 questions and annotated answers provides yet another vehicle to prepare students and life-long learners for subspecialty certification and for a deeper understanding of the field of psychosomatic medicine.

Theodore A. Stern, MD, FAPM

Questions

1. The former director of the Psychiatric Education Branch of the National Institute of Mental Health (NIMH), who provided support and encouragement in establishing consultation-liaison (C-L) programs throughout the United States, was:

   a. James Eaton
   b. William Herman
   c. James Jackson Putnam
   d. Howard Means
   e. Thomas Hackett

   _____

2. Classic studies on grief based on work with victims of the 1942 Coconut Grove fire in Boston were conducted by:

   a. Greta Bibring
   b. Helena Deutsch
   c. Erich Lindemann
   d. Thomas Hackett
   e. Avery Weisman

   _____

For questions 3-7 match the name in the left-hand column with the work or concept listed in the right-hand column.

3. _____ Broca

4. _____ Papez

5. _____ MacLean

6. _____ Nauta

7. _____ Laborgne

a. A neuroanatomist and author of a classic paper entitled "A Proposed Mechanism of Emotion"

b. A patient with aphasia found to have a softened area in the left frontal cortex

c. A neuroanatomist whose meticulous work delineated and expanded the concept of the limbic system

d. A French surgeon who wrote a 113-page monograph on the comparative neuroanatomy of mammals

e. Author of "Some psychiatric implications of physiological studies on the frontotemporal portion of the limbic system (visceral brain)"

Questions 8-9 are **true-false** questions.

8. Brodmann is known for his work on "split-brain" subjects that had corpus callosotomies for intractable epilepsy.

   _____

9. According to Dr. George Murray, a psychiatrist at the Massachusetts General Hospital, a smile is the limbic reaction of reality before it is fully understood by the neocortex (intellect).

   _____

10. The limbic system is involved with each of the following functions *except:*

    a. Attention
    b. Emotion
    c. Memory
    d. Bonding
    e. Vision

    ———

11. Which of the following structures is *not* thought to be part of the limbic system:

    a. Anterior nucleus of the thalamus
    b. Hippocampus
    c. Amygdala
    d. Mamillary bodies
    e. Brodmann's area 17

    ———

12. Each of the following factors is characteristic of "good copers" *except:*

    a. They tend to be optimistic, and they generally maintain a high level of morale.
    b. They tend to be practical.
    c. They tend to be resourceful.
    d. They tend not to be aware of emotional states.
    e. They tend to be open to suggestions.

    ———

13. Each of the following factors is characteristic of "bad copers" *except:*

    a. They tend to be reluctant to compromise or to ask for help.
    b. They tend to be intolerant of others.
    c. They tend to initiate corrective actions on their own behalf.

    d. They tend towards excessive denial or rationalization.
    e. They tend to be impulsive.

    ———

14. *True-false.* Courage requires an awareness of risk and is accompanied by an awareness of vulnerability.

    ———

15. The *most* common reason for psychiatric hospitalization is:

    a. Schizophrenia
    b. Depression
    c. Anxiety disorders
    d. Substance abuse
    e. Pain

    ———

Questions 16-42 are true-false questions.

16. Major depression in a man with terminal cancer is an appropriate reaction to his diagnosis.

    ———

17. Depression in the medically ill is diagnosed by application of the same criteria as found in the nonmedically ill.

    ———

18. Major depression increases the risk of cardiovascular dysfunction.

    ———

19. If left untreated, major depression has a natural course that is longer than that of minor depression.

    ———

20. Aprosodia following stroke typically results in major depression.

   _____

21. The presence of dementia of the Alzheimer's type does not increase the vulnerability to depression.

   _____

22. The sedative potency of available antidepressants in general is predicted by their in vitro affinity for the histamine H_1 receptor.

   _____

23. The propensity of available antidepressants to cause weight gain may be predicted by their in vitro affinity for the histamine H_1 receptor.

   _____

24. Diphenhydramine is a more potent antihistamine than is doxepin.

   _____

25. Amitriptyline has a greater affinity for muscarinic receptors than does protriptyline.

   _____

26. Orthostatic hypotension is directly related to each drug's in vitro affinity for the α_1-noradrenergic receptor.

   _____

27. In general, tertiary amine tricyclic antidepressants (TCAs) cause more orthostatic hypotension than do secondary amine TCAs.

   _____

28. A pretreatment fall of 10 mm Hg or greater in blood pressure predicts a good response to antidepressant medication in elderly patients.

   _____

29. Sinus tachycardia may result from the effect of a blockade of serotonin receptors on the vagal tone of the heart.

   _____

30. Tertiary amine TCAs typically cause sinus tachycardia in patients following cardiac transplantation.

   _____

31. Psychostimulants typically interfere with the appetite of depressed, medically ill, patients.

   _____

32. T-wave flattening occurs in fewer than 10% of lithium-treated patients.

   _____

33. For every completed suicide, approximately 18 to 20 attempts are made.

   _____

34. Drug overdose is the most common method of committing suicide for both men and women in the United States.

_____

35. Drug ingestion accounts for roughly two-thirds of unsuccessful suicides.

_____

36. The elderly are more likely to commit suicide than are younger individuals.

_____

37. One of every eight to 10 attempts in the elderly results in a completed suicide.

_____

38. Women are eight times more likely than men to complete suicide.

_____

39. Native Americans have a higher suicide rate than African Americans in the United States.

_____

40. Nearly 20% of people who complete suicide are legally intoxicated at the time of their death.

_____

41. Patients with AIDS have a suicide rate 10 times that of the general population.

_____

42. Head trauma is not associated with an increased risk of suicide.

_____

43. Each of the following conditions is associated with an increased risk of suicide *except:*

   a. Hypertension
   b. Spinal cord injury
   c. Sarcoid
   d. Cushing's disease
   e. Chronic renal failure.

_____

Questions 44-46 are true-false questions.

44. When the patient who is being evaluated for suicide refuses to allow the evaluating physician to contact family or friends, the clinician should not attempt to contact them.

_____

45. During the evaluation of suicide, the patient's safety must be assured until the patient is no longer at imminent risk of suicide.

_____

46. A patient should be hospitalized for further evaluation and treatment when the clinician cannot be reasonably certain that the patient is not at imminent risk of suicide.

_____

47. Each of the following conditions is an indication for ECT *except:*

    a. Depression
    b. Psychotic illness
    c. Posttraumatic stress disorder
    d. Mania
    e. Catatonia

    —————

48. *True-false.* Transient bradycardia and hypotension are rare following ECT.

    —————

49. The cardiac condition **least** likely to worsen with ECT is:

    a. Ischemic heart disease
    b. Hypertension
    c. Congestive heart failure
    d. Cardiac arrhythmias
    e. Cardiomyopathy

    —————

Questions 50-52 are true-false questions.

50. Parkinson's disease may improve with ECT.

    —————

51. ECT is contraindicated in pregnant women.

    —————

52. It is useful to premedicate the patient undergoing ECT with a benzodiazepine.

    —————

53. The routine pre-ECT work-up usually includes a thorough medical history, a physical examination, and each of the following tests *except:*

    a. A chest x-ray (CXR)
    b. An electrocardiogram (ECG)
    c. A complete blood count (CBC)
    d. An erythrocyte sedimentation rate (ESR)
    e. Serum electrolytes

    —————

Questions 54 and 55 are true-false questions.

54. Pulse oximetry and cardiac monitoring are advised in all patients undergoing general anesthesia.

    —————

55. Either atropine or glycopyrrolate are routinely administered during ECT because they decrease oral secretions.

    —————

56. Use of β-blockers effectively reduces the stress on the heart during ECT and attenuates each of the following *except:*

    a. Hypertension
    b. Congestive heart failure (CHF)
    c. Tachycardia
    d. Ectopy
    e. Cardiac ischemia

    —————

Questions 57-59 are true-false questions.

57. For most patients, a unilateral ECT stimulus is as effective as a bilateral stimulus.

    —————

58. Using a sine-wave stimulus is the standard of practice for ECT in the United States.

_____

59. Generalization of the seizure to the entire brain is essential for efficacy of ECT.

_____

60. Confusion that develops following ECT is associated with each of the following *except*

a. Pregnancy
b. High-stimulus intensity
c. Inadequate oxygenation
d. Prolonged seizure activity
e. Bilateral electrode placement

_____

61. The essential feature of delirium, according to the Diagnostic and Statistical Manual, Fourth Edition (DSM-IV), is a disturbance of consciousness accompanied by which of the following:

a. Anxiety
b. Depression with delusional features
c. Cognitive deficits not accounted for by past or evolving dementia
d. Depression with cognitive impairment
e. Agitation

_____

*Questions 62-65 are **true-false** questions.*

62. DSM-IV makes no distinction between a delirious patient with agitation or lethargy when it comes to diagnostic criteria.

_____

63. Sensory deprivation in the intensive care unit is a common cause of delirium.

_____

64. Patients with an adrenergic delirium typically present with dry skin and tachycardia.

_____

65. Physostigmine may be used as a diagnostic and therapeutic agent for cases of anticholinergic toxicity with delirium.

_____

66. Each of the following conditions *except* one should be assessed as causes for a delirious state because failure to promptly make a diagnosis and institute treatment may result in permanent central nervous system (CNS) damage.

a. Wernicke's disease
b. Hypoxia
c. Acute renal failure
d. Hypoglycemia
e. Hypertensive encephalopathy

_____

*Questions 67 and 68 are **true-false** questions.*

67. Bacteremia commonly causes an alteration in mental state.

_____

68. A score of less than 16 on the Mini-Mental State Examination (MMSE) of Folstein et al, is diagnostic of delirium.

_____

69. Frontal lobe function is **least** well assessed by observing for:

    a. A grasp reflex
    b. A snout response
    c. A palmomental reflex
    d. Pronater drift
    e. A glabellar response

    ———

*Questions 70 and 71 are **true-false** questions.*

70. When a patient performs the task of serial 7s, registration and memory are primarily being tested.

    ———

71. Delirious patients require use of a neuroleptic to control agitation and hallucinations.

    ———

72. When delirium with myoclonus develops, it is **most** likely secondary to which of the following:

    a. Digoxin
    b. Theophylline
    c. Atropine
    d. Meperidine
    e. Lorazepam

    ———

*Questions 73 and 74 are **true-false** questions.*

73. Haloperidol has not been approved by the Food and Drug Administration (FDA) for intravenous (IV) administration.

    ———

74. IV haloperidol may precipitate when infused through IV lines through which phenytoin or heparin is being administered.

    ———

Questions 75-79 involve matching the class of medication in the left-hand column with the antidote in the right-hand column.

75. ___ Benzodiazepines   a. Physostigmine

76. ___ Narcotics   b. Flumazenil

77. ___ Anticholinergics   c. Atropine

78. ___ Neuroleptics   d. Benztropine

79. ___ Cholinergics   e. Naloxone

*Questions 80-89 are **true-false** questions.*

80. A side-effect of the administration of physostigmine is seizures.

    ———

81. Excessive cholinergic reactions associated with physostigmine use can be prevented by preceding the injection by an IV injection of 0.2 mg of glycopyrrolate.

    ———

82. IV diazepam is more rapidly acting than IV haloperidol when used to treat agitated patients.

———

83. Akathisia and dystonia associated with IV haloperidol use is more common than with intramuscular (IM) haloperidol use.

———

84. Use of IV haloperidol has been associated with torsades de pointes.

———

85. Droperidol, a butyrophenone, is more sedating than is haloperidol.

———

86. Patients with Human immunodeficiency virus (HIV)-infection are more susceptible to extrapyramidal side effects of neuroleptics than are those without HIV infection.

———

87. One complication of propofol, a drug used for the sedation of critically ill patients, is a fat overload syndrome.

———

88. Administration of flumazenil to a narcotic-dependent patient can precipitate seizures.

———

89. It is not possible to assess the mental status of a chemically-paralyzed patient in the ICU.

———

90. Which of the following features is *not* characteristic of delirium?

   a. Abrupt onset
   b. Difficulty with attention with disturbed consciousness
   c. Positive family history
   d. Poor registration
   e. Dysgraphia

———

91. Which of the following features is *not* characteristic of dementia of the Alzheimer's type (DAT)?

   a. Insidious onset
   b. Gradually progressive over years
   c. Family history which may be positive for DAT
   d. Remote memory which is worse than recent memory
   e. Verbal and/or spatial memory deficits

———

92. Which of the following features is *not* characteristic of depression?

   a. Dysphoric mood
   b. Family history positive for depression
   c. Inconsistent memory
   d. Reduced speech latency
   e. Memory complaints present

———

93. Approximately what percent of the population more than 65 years of age suffers from some form of dementia?
   a. 5
   b. 10
   c. 15
   d. 20
   e. 25

———

*Questions 94-97 are **true-false** questions.*

94. Cognitive impairment, in the absence of significant impairment in social or occupational function or a significant decline from a prior level of function, does not meet criteria for a diagnosis of Alzheimer's disease.

   _____

95. When a patient has DAT, the individual lacks the ability to consent to procedures in the hospital setting.

   _____

96. DAT has a rate of cognitive decline roughly the same as that for Creutzfeldt-Jakob disease (CJD).

   _____

97. Incontinence, ataxia, and confusion are typically present in Binswanger's encephalopathy.

   _____

98. Vascular dementia is typically associated with each of the following *except*:

   a. Abrupt onset
   b. Step-wise deterioration
   c. Relative preservation of personality
   d. Diffuse neurological signs
   e. History of hypertension

   _____

*Questions 99-101 are **true-false** questions.*

99. Auditory hallucinations are more common than are visual hallucinations in DAT.

   _____

100. When a demented patient believes that their spouse is an impostor, the eponym Anton's syndrome is used.

   _____

101. With an apraxia, the patient is unable to recognize a familiar object despite intact sensory function.

   _____

Questions 102-106 involve matching the term in the left-hand column with the definition in the right-hand column.

102. _____ Hallucinations

103. _____ Delusions

104. _____ Illusions

105. _____ Thought disorder

106. _____ Akathisia

a. A misperception of a stimulus

b. A disruption in the form or organization of thinking

c. Sensory perceptions in the absence of any external source

d. Firmly-held false beliefs

e. An unpleasant sensation of motor restlessness or the inability to sit still

107. Wilson's disease may present with psychosis and each of the following findings **except**:

    a. Dysarthria
    b. Tremor
    c. Kayser Fleisher rings
    d. Paresis
    e. Gait disturbance

    ———

108. **True-false.** To meet criteria for schizophrenia, a patient must have demonstrated a decline in functioning and displayed either bizarre delusions or auditory hallucinations for at least 2 weeks.

    ———

109. Which of the following is the side effect **least** likely to be associated with treatment with thioridazine?

    a. Orthostatic hypotension
    b. Dystonia
    c. Tachycardia
    d. Sedation
    e. Weight gain

    ———

110. **True-false.** Risperidone is less anticholinergic than clozapine.

    ———

111. Which of the following side effects is **least** likely to occur with clozapine?

    a. Orthostatic hypotension
    b. Weight loss
    c. Tachycardia
    d. Sialorrhea
    e. Seizures

    ———

112. **True-false**. A dangerous side effect of clozapine treatment that has led to routine laboratory testing is leukocytosis.

    ———

113. Antipsychotic-induced Parkinsonian side effects improve with each of the following **except:**

    a. Reduction in the neuroleptic dose
    b. Addition of benztropine
    c. Change to a higher-potency neuroleptic
    d. Addition of amantadine
    e. Addition of a β-blocker.

    ———

114. **True-false.** Tardive dyskinesia rarely occurs less than six months into treatment with a neuroleptic.

    ———

115. Each of the following is a sign of neuroleptic malignant syndrome **except:**

    a. Hyperthermia
    b. Rigidity
    c. Increased creatine phosphokinase (CPK)
    d. Leukopenia
    e. Autonomic instability

    ———

*Questions 116 and 117 are **true-false** questions.*

116. Patients with a history of malignant hyperthermia are at higher risk of developing neuroleptic malignant syndrome.

    ———

117. Most antipsychotic drugs are metabolized by the 3A4 isoenzyme system.

    _____

118. Signs and symptoms of polydipsia include each of the following *except:*

    a. Hyponatremia
    b. Nausea
    c. Blurred vision
    d. Lethargy
    e. Palpitations

    _____

119. Which of the following populations has the *highest* reported prevalence of panic disorder?

    a. Patients in the primary care setting
    b. Patients in cardiology practices
    c. Patients in pediatric practices
    d. Patients in the general population
    e. Patients in a geriatric practice

    _____

120. The locus coeruleus (LC) is the primary source of the brain's:

    a. Serotonin
    b. Norepinephrine
    c. γ-Aminobutyric acid (GABA)
    d. Acetylcholine
    e. Glutamate

    _____

121. Each of the following features suggests an organically based anxiety syndrome *except:*

    a. A negative childhood history of anxiety symptoms
    b. An onset of anxiety symptoms after the age of 35 years
    c. A lack of a personal or family history of anxiety disorders
    d. Presence of depressive symptoms
    e. A lack of avoidance behavior

    _____

*Questions 122-141 are **true-false** questions.*

122. Less than 50% of patients with panic disorder present with somatic complaints.

    _____

123. Mitral valve prolapse is associated with panic disorder.

    _____

124. Major depression occurs in roughly one-third of patients with panic disorder.

    _____

125. Selective serotonin-reuptake inhibitors (SSRIs) have become a first-line treatment for panic disorder, as well as for other anxiety disorders.

    _____

126. SSRI treatment of panic-disordered patients should begin with one-half the usual starting dose.

    _____

127. The onset of the benefit of SSRIs for panic disorder usually begins within the first week.

_____

128. Most patients with panic disorder treated with alprazolam respond to doses of 1 to 2 mg qd.

_____

129. The half-life of clonazepam is roughly equivalent to that of alprazolam.

_____

130. Midazolam is commonly used to treat panic disorder and post-traumatic stress disorder among medically ill patients.

_____

131. Buspirone is a low-potency benzodiazepine with proven anti-panic efficacy and efficacy for generalized anxiety disorder.

_____

132. Even a single, brief, and detailed discussion by a physician yields measurable reductions in alcoholism's consequences.

_____

133. Alcohol is a GABA antagonist.

_____

134. Unsuccessful interviews of intoxicated patients in emergency rooms tend to instantly attempt to make the drunk person civil.

_____

135. Sustained eye contact should be made with an intoxicated patient.

_____

136. In pathologic intoxication, hallucinations typically develop for which he/she is usually amnestic.

_____

137. Alcohol withdrawal seizures typically occur 3-5 days after the stoppage of heavy drinking.

_____

138. Alcoholic hallucinosis occurs in a patient with a clear sensorium.

_____

139. Alcohol withdrawal seizures are estimated to occur in 5% to 7% of unmedicated withdrawing alcoholics.

_____

140. Wernicke's encephalopathy is characterized by confabulation.

_____

141. Korsakoff's psychosis tends to improve.

_____

142. Wernicke's encephalopathy is characterized by each of the following *except:*
    a. Ataxia
    b. Dysarthria
    c. Nystagmus
    d. Global confusion
    e. Exhaustion

_____

143. **True-false.** Folic acid should be administered to the patient with suspected Wernicke's encephalopathy to prevent the development of an irreversible and incapacitating amnestic disorder.

_____

144. Disulfiram interactions with alcohol result in each of the following **except:**

a. Hypotension
b. Headache
c. Bradycardia
d. Nausea
e. Vomiting

_____

145. Signs and symptoms of acute cocaine intoxication are similar to those of intoxication with which of the following?

a. Benzodiazepines
b. Narcotics
c. Amphetamines
d. Anticholinergics
e. LSD

_____

146. Typical complaints associated with acute cocaine intoxication include each of the following **except:**

a. Anorexia
b. Miosis
c. Insomnia
d. Hyperactivity
e. Rapid speech

_____

147. Typically, chronic cocaine use produces each of the following **except:**

a. Psychological dependency
b. Tolerance
c. Irritability
d. Euphoria
e. Anxiety

_____

148. Signs of opiate withdrawal include each of the following **except:**

a. Sweating
b. Yawning
c. Miosis
d. Lacrimation
e. Rhinorrhea.

_____

149. Signs of severe opiate withdrawal include each of the following **except:**

a. Tachycardia
b. Vomiting
c. Hypertension
d. Hypersomnia
e. Abdominal cramps

_____

150. Buprenorphine is:

a. A short-acting partial opiate agonist
b. A long-acting partial opiate agonist
c. A short-acting opiate antagonist
d. A long-acting opiate antagonist
e. Another name for Narcan

_____

151. Which of the following statements about clonidine is *not* true?

    a. It suppresses the autonomic symptoms of narcotic withdrawal.
    b. It can be associated with hypotension.
    c. It should be used in doses no higher than 0.6 mg qd or 0.2 mg tid.
    d. It can be associated with sedation.
    e. It is an α_2-adrenergic antagonist.

    _____

152. When a patient who has used benzodiazepines chronically suddenly discontinues using them, withdrawal symptoms typically include each of the following *except:*

    a. Anxiety
    b. Euphoria
    c. Insomnia
    d. Irritability
    e. Seizures

    _____

153. *True-false.* Flumazenil can precipitate seizures in a patient taking tricyclic antidepressants.

    _____

154. The typical pupillary reaction to barbiturate overdose includes *which* of the following?

    a. No change in pupillary size
    b. Pinpoint pupils
    c. Fixed and dilated pupils
    d. Unequal pupils
    e. Mid-position fixed pupils

    _____

155. Cross tolerance exists between barbiturates and *which* of the following agents?

    a. Narcotics
    b. Anticholinergics
    c. Benzodiazepines
    d. Neuroleptics
    e. Antihistamines

    _____

156. Treatment of barbiturate overdose may include each of the following *except:*

    a. Maintenance of an adequate airway
    b. Diuresis
    c. Acidification of the urine
    d. Dialysis
    e. Charcoal resin hemoperfusion.

    _____

157. *True-false.* A 30 mg oral dose of phenobarbital is roughly equivalent to a 100 mg oral dose of pentobarbital.

    _____

158. Which of the following is a self-rating scale used to screen for psychiatric disorders?

    a. Hamilton Rating Scale for Depression
    b. Brief Psychiatric Rating Scale
    c. Beck Depression Inventory
    d. Yale-Brown Obsessive-Compulsive Scale
    e. Young Mania Scale

    _____

*Questions 159-169 are **true-false** questions.*

159. The Global Assessment of Function (GAF) Scale is a routine part of the DSM-IV multi-axial assessment registered on Axis IV.

_____

160. The GAF provides a composite index of symptoms and dimensions pertaining to quality of life.

_____

161. An understanding that a patient's condition is influenced by psychosocial factors implies that psychotropic medications should be withheld.

_____

162. Discussions preceding the initiation of psychotropic medications should include target symptoms, the anticipated time course of response to treatment, the anticipated length of treatment, and the strategies available to react to side effects, or lack of efficacy.

_____

163. When discussing decisions regarding choice of a particular psychotropic medication with a patient, consideration of the cost of the medication is of little relevance.

_____

164. In fewer than one-half of patients with major psychiatric disorders, initiation of a psychotropic brings about significant improvement despite accurate diagnosis.

_____

165. Apparent treatment refractoriness is often the result of prescription of inadequate doses or to patient non-compliance.

_____

166. Pharmacodynamic processes refer to absorption, distribution, metabolism, and excretion; these are factors that determine plasma levels and the local availability of the drug to biologically active sites.

_____

167. Factors that speed gastric emptying or diminish intestinal motility may increase plasma drug concentrations.

_____

168. Antacids may form complexes with psychotropics, allowing them to pass unabsorbed through the GI lumen.

_____

169. Lithium is a fat-soluble drug.

_____

170. Each of the following drugs is highly protein bound, that is, greater than 90% exists in the bound form in plasma, *except:*

    a. Fluoxetine
    b. Amitriptyline
    c. Diazepam
    d. Haloperidol
    e. Gabapentin

_____

171. Hepatic metabolism can be induced by each of the following *except:*

    a. Barbiturates
    b. Cimetidine
    c. Rifampin
    d. Phenytoin
    e. Cigarettes

    ———

172. Common inhibitors of hepatic metabolism include each of the following *except:*

    a. Ketoconazole
    b. Erythromycin
    c. Phenobarbital
    d. Propranolol
    e. Fluoxetine

    ———

173. Increased serum levels of lithium are likely to result from each of the following *except:*

    a. Reduced glomerular filtration rate
    b. Use of thiazide diuretics
    c. Use of theophylline
    d. Dehydration
    e. Increased proximal tubular reabsorption of lithium

    ———

*Questions 174-177 are **true-false** questions.*

174. Alkalinization of the urine increases the rate of excretion of weak bases, such as amphetamines and phencyclidine (PCP).

    ———

175. Acidification of the urine may be achieved through use of ascorbic acid or ammonium chloride.

    ———

176. Alkalinization of the urine by means of sodium bicarbonate may promote the excretion of weak acids, including phenobarbital.

    ———

177. Gabapentin is primarily hepatically metabolized.

    ———

178. Which of the following neuroleptics is *not* highly protein bound?

    a. Thioridazine
    b. Molindone
    c. Haloperidol
    d. Perphenazine
    e. Thiothixene

    ———

*Questions 179-182 are **true-false** questions.*

179. Risperidone is a high-potency neuroleptic with a high affinity for α_1-adrenergic receptors and a tendency to produce orthostatic hypotension.

    ———

180. Addition of antacids to neuroleptics may lower serum levels of neuroleptic agents.

    ———

181. Smoking cigarettes will decrease antipsychotic drug plasma levels.

    ———

182. Addition of an SSRI to a neuroleptic will decrease the level of the neuroleptic agent.

_____

183. Which of the following agents would *not* be expected to increase lithium levels?

a. Aminophylline
b. Nonsteroidal antiinflammatory drugs
c. Tetracycline
d. Thiazide diuretics
e. Metronidazole

_____

184. *True-false.* Co-administration of lithium and succinylcholine prolongs muscle paralysis.

_____

185. Which of the following statements about lithium is *not* true?

a. Lithium is completely absorbed in the GI tract.
b. Lithium distributes throughout total body water.
c. Peak concentrations of lithium are reached in less than 2 hours with standard preparations.
d. 95% of lithium is excreted in the urine.
e. Lithium is highly bound to plasma proteins.

_____

186. Which of the following statements about valproic acid is *not* true?

a. It is rapidly absorbed after oral administration.
b. It is 80% to 95% protein bound.
c. It has an elimination half-life of 18-20 hours.
d. Clearance is essentially unchanged in those with renal disease.
e. Clearance is essentially unchanged in the elderly.

_____

187. Which of the following statements about valproic acid is *not* true?

a. It inhibits hepatic isoenzymes.
b. It tends to inhibit oxidative reactions.
c. It inhibits the metabolism of carbamazepine.
d. It displaces carbamazepine from protein-binding sites.
e. It causes a doubling of lamotrigine levels.

_____

*Questions 188 and 189 are **true-false** questions.*

188. Addition of cimetidine to valproic acid leads to decreased clearance of valproic acid.

_____

189. Addition of fluoxetine to valproic acid may result in valproic acid toxicity.

_____

190. Which of the following statements about carbamazepine is *not* true?

    a. It is structurally related to the tricyclic antidepressant, imipramine.
    b. It is slowly absorbed from the GI tract.
    c. Its levels are lowered by addition of erythromycin.
    d. It is only moderately protein bound, that is, 60% to 85%.
    e. It is a potent inducer of hepatic metabolism.

    _____

191. Which of the following statements about tricyclic antidepressants is *not* true?

    a. They inhibit the presynaptic neuronal uptake of norepinephrine and serotonin.
    b. They have quinidine-like effects on cardiac conduction.
    c. They have significant anticholinergic activity.
    d. They are highly protein-bound.
    e. They are poorly absorbed from the GI tract.

    _____

192. Tricyclic antidepressants with two methyl groups on the terminal nitrogen of the tricyclic side chain include each of the following *except:*

    a. Amitriptyline
    b. Doxepin
    c. Clomipramine
    d. Protriptyline
    e. Trimipramine

    _____

*Questions 193-202 are **true-false** questions.*

193. Addition of carbamazepine to a tricyclic antidepressant can decrease tricyclic antidepressant levels.

    _____

194. Tricyclic antidepressants can antagonize the antihypertensive effects of guanethidine or clonidine by interference of neuronal uptake by noradrenergic neurons.

    _____

195. Hypoglycemia may result from co-administration of secondary or tertiary amine TCAs and sulfonylurea-hypoglycemic agents.

    _____

196. Co-administration of tricyclic antidepressants and cimetidine or methylphenidate can raise tricyclic antidepressant levels.

    _____

197. Paroxetine is more highly protein-bound than is venlafaxine.

    _____

198. Among the SSRIs, only venlafaxine appears to be a potent inhibitor of P450 1A2 isoenzymes.

    _____

199. Intestinal monoamine oxidase (MAO) is predominantly MAO-B, whereas MAO in the brain is predominantly MAO-A.

    _____

200. Both phenelzine and tranylcypromine are nonspecific inhibitors of MAO-A and MAO-B.

_____

201. Inhibition of MAO by phenelzine is irreversible, and restoration of enzyme activity after phenelzine is discontinued takes up to 2 weeks.

_____

202. Treatment of an MAO inhibitor (MAOI)-associated hypertensive crisis involves use of an α_1-adrenergic antagonist.

_____

203. Which of the following agents is the *least* likely to cause a hypertensive crisis when co-administered with an MAOI?

    a. L-dopa
    b. Nifedipine
    c. Amphetamine
    d. Phentermine
    e. Pseudoephedrine

_____

204. Which of the following agents is *most* likely to cause a hypertensive reaction when co-administered with an MAOI?

    a. Methylphenidate
    b. Norepinephrine
    c. Isoproterenol
    d. Ephedrine
    e. Phentolamine

_____

205. Which of the following factors is *least* likely to produce a hypertensive reaction when co-administered with an MAOI?

    a. Cheddar cheese
    b. Cream cheese
    c. Salami
    d. Sauerkraut
    e. Imported beer

_____

206. A dangerous interaction is *most* likely to occur with MAOIs and which of the following agents?

    a. Propoxyphene
    b. Codeine
    c. Morphine
    d. Meperidine
    e. Oxycodone

_____

207. Management of Parkinsonism side effects can be achieved with each of the following *except:*

    a. Amantadine
    b. Benztropine
    c. Diphenhydramine
    d. Metoclopramide
    e. Biperiden

_____

208. Pharmacological treatment of orthostatic hypotension secondary to antidepressants may involve each of the following *except:*

    a. Caffeine
    b. Clonidine
    c. Fludrocortisone
    d. Salt tablets
    e. T-3

_____

209. Sexual dysfunction secondary to SSRIs may be treated by each of the following agents *except:*

    a. Bupropion
    b. Cyproheptadine
    c. Bethanechol
    d. Clonidine
    e. Yohimbine

    —————

210. Which of the following statements about clonidine is *least* likely to be true?

    a. It is highly lipophilic and readily crosses the blood-brain barrier.
    b. It stimulates α_2-adrenergic receptors.
    c. It can successfully treat Tourette's syndrome, as well as motor and phonic tics.
    d. It can cause or exacerbate akathisia.
    e. It can suppress signs and symptoms of narcotic withdrawal.

    —————

Questions 211-215 involve matching the condition in the left-hand column with the corresponding statement in the right-hand column.

211. ——— Malingering

212. ——— Factitious disorders

213. ——— Somatization disorder

214. ——— Hypo-chondriasis

215. ——— Conversion disorder

a. Involves a loss or change in sensory function suggestive of a physical disorder but caused by psychological problems

b. A chronic syndrome of recurring multiple somatic symptoms not explainable medically and associated with psychological distress.

c. False or exaggerated symptoms are reported for clear-cut secondary gain.

d. Simulated or feigned illness without apparent self-advantage

e. A preoccupation with the fear or belief of having a serious disease based upon the misinterpretation of benign physical signs or sensations as evidence of disease

216. Malingering should be suspected by the presence of each of the following symptoms or features *except:*

    a. A medical legal case and referral by an attorney
    b. When the individual enjoys fooling physicians

    c. A marked discrepancy between apparent distress or disability and objective findings
    d. A lack of cooperation with the diagnostic work-up and treatment plan
    e. The presence of an antisocial personality disorder

    —————

217. Each of the following features is characteristic of factitious disorder *except:*

    a. A high percentage of successful psychiatric referrals
    b. A facility for lying and fooling physicians
    c. A driven quality to create signs and symptoms over and over again
    d. The presence of pseudologia fantastica
    e. Extensive knowledge about medical conditions

    ―――――

218. *True-false.* Patients with factitious disorder always feign or simulate medical and surgical complaints.

    ―――――

219. The term Münchausen syndrome was first used and reported in a 1951 Lancet article by:

    a. Peter Reich
    b. Marvin Stern
    c. Richard Asher
    d. Charles Ford
    e. Arthur Barsky

    ―――――

Questions 220-224 are true-false questions.

220. Conversion symptoms are intentionally produced or feigned.

    ―――――

221. Patients with monosymptomatic hypochondriacal psychosis have a single fixed belief that one is diseased.

    ―――――

222. The formal diagnosis of chronic fatigue syndrome requires exclusion of common psychiatric disorders.

    ―――――

223. Fibromyalgia is a syndrome of generalized muscle pain and tenderness at specific trigger points.

    ―――――

224. Criteria for irritable bowel syndrome include each of the following: continuous or recurrent abdominal pain or discomfort relieved by defecation for at least 3 months and associated with a change in stool frequency or consistency; that is, altered stool frequency, watery stool, a sense of straining or urgency, and the feeling of incomplete evacuation, passage of mucous, bloating, or feelings of abdominal distention.

    ―――――

For questions 225-227, match the conditions in the left-hand column with the characteristics for those conditions in the right-hand column.

225. _____ Antisocial personality disorder

226. _____ Borderline personality disorder

227. _____ Narcissistic personality disorder

a. A pattern of grandiosity, need for admiration, and lack of empathy

b. A pattern of instability of interpersonal relationships, self-image, and affect, as well as marked impulsivity

c. A pattern of disregard for, and violation of, the rights of others

*Questions 228 and 229 are **true-false** questions.*

228. In limit-setting confrontations with manipulative, entitled patients, the consultant usually needs to model firmness for staff and appeal to the patient's sense of entitlement.

_____

229. Dependent, manipulative patients stir up a sense of omnipotence in caregivers.

_____

230. Which of the following psychological defenses is **least** likely to lead to problems in a patient with a borderline personality?

a. Splitting
b. Psychotic denial
c. Rationalization
d. Projective identification
e. Dissociation

_____

*Questions 231 and 232 are **true-false** questions.*

231. Projective identification is a distinct, rigid separation of positive and negative thoughts or feelings.

_____

232. Primitive idealization is the tendency to see some staff as totally good to protect the patient from the bad staff or from the patient's medical condition.

_____

233. Which of the following statements is **least** important about the management of difficult patients in the medical setting?
    a. Rapid evaluation of pressing psychiatric problems is key if the patient appears about to lose control of violent or self-destructive impulses.
    b. Differential diagnosis of the difficult patient, using a biopsychosocial approach, is crucial.
    c. Identification of patient/staff dissonance is best to establish a plan of action.
    d. The expertise of the consultant should be emphasized to patients and staff so credit can be duly attributed for a successful outcome.
    e. Treatment recommendations should address both psychological and psychopharmacological issues of the patient.

*Questions 234-236 are **true-false** questions.*

234. Education of the consultee and the staff can help to reduce dissonance regarding a difficult patient and lead to a conceptual framework for dealing with future difficult patients.

_____

235. Tactical brief therapy of the difficult patient is of value to contain affect by means of redefinition and redirection of self-defeating behavior.

_____

236. The International Association of the Study of Pain has defined pain as an unpleasant sensory experience caused by actual but not potential tissue damage.

_____

Questions 237-241 involve matching the term in the left-hand column with the definition or characteristics in the right-hand column.

237. _____ Nociceptive pain

238. _____ Allodynia

239. _____ Hypoesthesia

240. _____ Hyperpathia

241. _____ Hypoalgesia

a. Pain due to activation of a-delta or c-sensory fibers that responds to thermal, mechanical, or chemical stimuli

b. A heightened response that emerges after the offending stimulus is removed

c. A decreased sensitivity to pain

d. A pain caused by a noxious stimulus such as cold, vibration, or light mechanical touch

e. A decreased sensitivity to any stimulation

242. *True-false.* Major depressive disorder is diagnosed in approximately 50% of patients with chronic pain.

_____

243. The so-called conversion V, present among many patients with chronic pain, is detected by use of which of the following tests?

a. The SCL-90
b. The MMPI
c. The BPRS
d. The McGill Pain Inventory
e. The EMG

_____

Questions 244 and 245 are true-false questions.

244. A patient should not have his/her pain labeled as psychogenic pain merely because it is not understood, or because it is unresponsive to treatment.

_____

245. Positive responses to a placebo prove that pain is not real and that the patient will not benefit from an active medication.

_____

246. Roughly what percent of the general population are placebo responders?

a. Less than 5
b. 15-20
c. 25-30
d. 35-40
e. Greater than 50

_____

Questions 247 and 248 are true-false questions.

247. One of the clinical hazards of placebo use is that the patient may feel tricked if he/she discovers that a placebo had been administered without consent.

_____

248. Step 1 of the World Health Organization's three-step guidelines for pain management involves the use of nonsteroidal antiinflammatory drugs, aspirin, or codeine.

_____

249. Side effects of NSAIDs include each of the following *except:*

a. Bronchospasm in aspirin-sensitive patients
b. Gastric ulcers
c. Renal failure in association with angiotensin-converting enzymes (ACE) inhibitors
d. Lower blood pressure in patients treated with β-blockers and diuretics
e. Precipitation of lithium toxicity.

_____

Questions 250-252 are true-false questions.

250. Pentazocine is a mixed kappa and sigma receptor agonist and antagonist.

_____

251. Meperidine in its parenteral preparation is twice as potent as it is in its oral preparation.

_____

252. The active metabolite of meperidine has a short duration of action (4-6 hours) and can cause irritability and agitation.

_____

253. The active metabolite of meperidine (normeperidine) causes each of the following *except:*
    a. Auditory and visual hallucinations
    b. Paranoia
    c. Myoclonus
    d. Renal impairment
    e. Seizures

_____

Questions 254-264 are **true-false** *questions.*

254. Normeperidine toxicity is likely to occur when meperidine is given in doses of 300 mg or more intravenously per day for 3 or more days.

_____

255. Methadone's analgesic efficacy is 18 to 36 hours.

_____

256. Pentazocine and buprenorphine are opioids with mixed antagonist-agonist properties.

_____

257. The risk of opioid addiction in medically ill patients is approximately 1% to 2%.

_____

258. In the spinal cord, the anterolateral columns carry the serotonergic descending spinal pain pathways that modulate 80% of the spinal analgesic effects of opiates.

_____

259. Potent serotonin reuptake blocking is not essential to pain relief.

_____

260. Gabapentin is the only direct glutamate/aspartate antagonist in the United States that also inhibits sodium channels.

_____

261. Valproate, as opposed to carbamazepine, has little or no role in the treatment of pain conditions.

_____

262. Mexiletine is an agent used for the treatment of neuropathic pain.

_____

263. Sympathetically-mediated pain may respond to the use of phentolamine or clonidine.

_____

264. In the context of general hospitals, psychiatrists have positions with the legal authority to make decisions about competency and treatment refusal.

_____

265. To establish a claim of malpractice, a plaintiff must prove four things. Which of the following statements is **not** required for a claim of malpractice?
    a. It must be proved that the defendant physician owed a duty to the injured party.
    b. When the injured party is the patient, the duty is to perform up to the standards of physicians in the community practicing in that specialty.
    c. That the clinician failed to keep matters revealed by a patient from the ears of a third party.
    d. The negligent physician's behavior needs to be shown to have been the direct cause of the damages.
    e. The negligent behavior needs to be shown to have been the direct cause of the actual damages.

    _____

*Questions 266-282 are **true-false** questions.*

266. The Tarasoff vs the Board of Regents case held that psychotherapists have a duty to act to protect third parties where the therapist knows, or should have known, that the patient poses a threat of severe harm to the third party.

    _____

267. Liability can arise when medical or surgical colleagues fail to breech confidentiality and warn family members, or other contacts, about the potential for contagion from an infectious disease.

    _____

268. Abandonment is the unilateral severance of a relationship by a physician, leaving the patient without needed medical care.

    _____

269. A physician may not terminate the treatment relationship with a patient for failure to keep appointments.

    _____

270. When the physician terminates a treatment relationship, the physician should notify the patient of the decision, the available treatment options, and available sources of emergency care.

    _____

271. When a competent patient refuses life-saving medical treatment, the patient's decision should be over-ridden and treatment initiated.

    _____

272. Active steps taken by a physician to end a patient's life are considered to be a routine part of hospice care.

    _____

273. In 1990, the U.S. Supreme Court handed down an opinion in Cruzan vs Director, Missouri Department of Public Health and found that all competent individuals have a right to refuse life-sustaining treatment.

    _____

274. In 1990, the U.S. Supreme Court handed down an opinion in *Cruzan v. Director, Missouri Department of Public Health,* and found that, when a patient is incompetent, the court should decide the appropriate treatment of the individual.

_____

275. Under the Patient Self-Determination Act of 1990, all health care facilities, nursing homes, and health maintenance organizations must complete advance directives on their patients.

_____

276. Informed consent is only required before treatments or procedures likely to be associated with bodily harm or death.

_____

277. Informed consent is not required in an emergency in which the delay would seriously threaten the well being of the patient.

_____

278. Informed consent need not be obtained in cases where the information needed for consent would cause the patient's physical or mental health to deteriorate.

_____

279. When the amount of information to be provided to a patient is determined by what the patient would require to make an informed decision, it is known as the professional standard.

_____

280. The professional standard of informed consent is one in which the physician is required to give the amount of information that the average physician, in that specialty, would provide under similar circumstances.

_____

281. Informed consent requires that consent be given voluntarily.

_____

282. Only a judge can declare a person to be incompetent for specific functions or for all activities.

_____

283. Applebaum and Grisso suggested four criteria that should be covered when assessing decision-making capacity. Select the factor **not** necessary for assessment of decision-making capacity.
    a. Does the patient manifest a preference?
    b. Does the patient have a life-threatening condition?
    c. Is the patient capable of attaining the factual understanding of the situation?
    d. Does the patient have an appreciation of the significance of the facts presented?
    e. Is the patient able to use the information presented in a rational fashion to reach a decision?

*Questions 284-295 are **true-false** questions.*

284. Competency is an all or nothing proposition.

_____

285. The criteria for having capacity to make decisions for refusal of treatment are the same as those for treatment acceptance.

_____

286. A diagnosis of dementia confirms the labeling of a patient as incompetent.

_____

287. The psychiatric consultant asked to evaluate a patient threatening to leave against medical advice must evaluate whether the patient is competent to make that decision.

_____

288. For the hospitalized infant, the key developmental challenge is to maintain the quality of attachment between physician and child.

_____

289. The three phases of separation anxiety seen in infants, according to Bowlby, in the classic work on attachment, are protest, despair, and rapprochement.

_____

290. According to Bowlby, the stage of separation anxiety in an infant in which the infant acutely, vigorously, and loudly thrashes and attempts to prevent departure of the mother or rapidly attempts to recapture her is termed protest.

_____

291. According to Bowlby, the stage of separation anxiety in an infant in which the infant is less active, may cry in a monotone with less vigor, begins to withdraw and appears hopeless is termed despair.

_____

292. According to Bowlby, the stage of separation anxiety in an infant in which the infant seems more alert and accepting of nursing care is termed rapprochement.

_____

293. In the preschool phase (ages 2-1/2 to 6 years), magical thinking is often involved and invoked by a child to explain how things occur in the world.

_____

294. For the preschooler (ages 2-1/2 to 6 years), the child's perception is that all life events revolve around the family.

_____

295. A medically ill preschooler often envisions the body as a shell filled with blood, food, and stool, which can ooze out of any hole in the skin.

_____

296. Suspicion of child abuse should be raised when each of the following is present *except:*
    a. When bruises that resemble finger or hand prints are present
    b. When bruises appear on body surfaces that do not normally bear the brunt of accidental falls
    c. When a bruised child says he frequently goes skateboarding without a helmet or elbow pads
    d. When bruises are present in various stages of healing
    e. When bruises or fractures and accidents have occurred that are inconsistent with the caretaker's explanation

    _____

297. *True-false.* Neglect of children is the absence of adequate parenting that results in a child being inadequately supervised, fed, clothed, or emotionally attended to.

    _____

298. Manifestations in children of neglect by parents can be evidence by each of the following *except:*
    a. Failure to thrive
    b. The occurrence of preventable accidents
    c. Attention deficit hyperactivity disorder
    d. Dermatological conditions of poor hygiene
    e. Missed routine and specialty medical appointments

    _____

Questions 299-305 are true-false questions.

299. The incidence of sexual abuse is reported to be more than twice as common in girls as it is in boys.

    _____

300. A child who presents with a sexually transmitted disease should be suspected as having been sexually abused.

    _____

301. There is no single personality profile of a sexual abuse perpetrator.

    _____

302. Münchausen syndrome by proxy is a form of child abuse.

    _____

303. Except in emergency situations, consent must be obtained from the custodial parent or legal guardian before the use of any compounds in the pediatric population.

    _____

304. The FDA prohibits the use of drugs in other than approved uses.

    _____

305. The typical starting dose for pemoline for ADHD is 2.5 to 5 mg qd.

    _____

306. Which of the following statements about pemoline is **not** true?

    a. It may exacerbate tics in those with tics.
    b. It leads to a toxic psychosis when high doses are used.
    c. It should not be prescribed to those taking anticonvulsants.
    d. It may lead to choreoathetosis in 1% to 2%.
    e. It may lead to hepatitis in 1% to 2%.

    ———

307. Clonidine is used for each the following conditions **except:**

    a. Tourette's syndrome
    b. ADHD
    c. Enuresis
    d. Aggressiveness
    e. Sleep disturbance

    ———

308. Which of the following statements about clonidine is **not** true?

    a. It is an α-adrenergic agonist.
    b. Its half-life ranges from 5.5 hours to 8.5 hours in adults.
    c. Its primary use is in the treatment of hypertension.
    d. It is usually prescribed in daily doses of 3 to 10 mcg/kg in divided doses.
    e. Its use is contraindicated in patients with asthma.

    ———

309. Each of the following is commonly reported as a side effect associated with clonidine **except:**

    a. Hypotension
    b. Sedation
    c. Bradycardia
    d. Dry mouth
    e. Depression

    ———

*Questions 310-317 are **true-false** questions.*

310. Pregnancy is protective with respect to the emergence or persistence of psychiatric disorders.

    ———

311. Post-marketing surveillance data reveals higher rates of major congenital malformations than noted in the general population for sertraline, paroxetine, and venlafaxine.

    ———

312. The risk of cardiovascular malformation following prenatal exposure to lithium is approximately 1 in 500.

    ———

313. The risk of developing spina bifida is greater than that for developing neural tube deficits in association with use of valproic acid and carbamazepine.

    ———

314. Treatment of psychosis during pregnancy with haloperidol or thiothixene is problematic because of the risk of congenital malformations when used in the first trimester.

    ———

315. Use of lower potency neuroleptics, such as chlorpromazine, is associated with congenital malformations when compared to its use in non-neuroleptic-exposed women.

    ———

316. All psychotropics (including atypical antipsychotics, antidepressants, lithium, and benzodiazepines) are secreted into breast milk.

_____

317. Lithium is predictably secreted into breast milk with a concentration of approximately one-half of the maternal plasma level.

_____

318. Each of the following cohorts of women appear to have an increased risk of post-partum worsening of mood *except*:
    a. Women who deliver after the age of 35 years
    b. Women with a past history of major depressive disorder
    c. Women with bipolar disorder
    d. Women with major depressive disorder during pregnancy
    e. Women with a history of post-partum depression

_____

*Questions 319 - 327 are **true-false** questions.*

319. The prevalence of post-partum depression is approximately 5%.

_____

320. The half-life of lorazepam increases in patients with end-stage renal disease from approximately 10 to 20 hours to 30 to 70 hours.

_____

321. Less than one-third of cases of liver failure in the United States are caused by alcoholic cirrhosis or alcoholic hepatitis.

_____

322. All centers that perform organ transplantation in the United States use the same criteria for selection of donors and organ recipients.

_____

323. HIV infection is caused by the DNA virus HIV type I.

_____

324. The virus that causes AIDS causes disease by infecting cells of the immune system that have a CD-4 receptor on their surface.

_____

325. The progression of HIV infection causes a fall in CD-4 positive lymphocytes, which results in immunosuppression.

_____

326. When CD-4 lymphocyte counts fall below 600 per microliter, the risk for opportunistic infections is high.

_____

327. HIV infects the brain via macrophages that are infected in the periphery.

_____

328. Common neuropsychiatric side effects of zidovudine (AZT) include each of the *following* **except:**

    a. Headache
    b. Agitation
    c. Insomnia
    d. Hallucinations
    e. Mania

    _____

329. Common neuropsychiatric side effects of acyclovir include each of the following **except**:

    a. Visual hallucinations
    b. Depersonalization
    c. Confusion
    d. Hyperacusis
    e. Hypersomnia

    _____

*Questions 330 - 333 are **true-false** questions.*

330. In the hospitalized patient with asymptomatic HIV infection or a CD-4 count greater than 500, it is rare to have an underlying HIV-related condition as a source for delirium.

    _____

331. A sudden change in mental status is characteristic of AIDS dementia complex.

    _____

332. Patients with HIV dementia are at greater risk for neuroleptic-induced extrapyramidal side effects.

    _____

333. A diagnosis of AIDS-dementia complex implies that a patient is incompetent.

    _____

334. According to the American Academy of Neurology, which of the following is **not** a feature of HIV-associated cognitive motor complex?

    a. An acquired abnormality in attention
    b. Cognitive dysfunction causing impairment at work
    c. Evidence of CNS lymphoma
    d. An absence of clouding of consciousness
    e. A decline in motivation or emotional control

    _____

*Questions 335-336 are **true-false** questions.*

335. Trail Making A and B Tests primarily test visual-spatial function.

    _____

336. Due to the prevalence of HIV-related dementia in HIV-infected patients, psychostimulants are contraindicated.

    _____

337. Likely causes for secondary mania in HIV-infected patients with CD-4 counts less than 100 per microliter, include each of the following **except**:

    a. Toxoplasmosis
    b. Cryptococcal meningitis
    c. Meningioma
    d. Non-Hodgkin's lymphoma
    e. Use of didanosine (DDI)

    _____

*Questions 338-340 are **true-false** questions.*

338. Major depressive disorder is a normal consequence of HIV-1 disease.

   _____

339. Peripheral neuropathy affects up to 15% of patients with AIDS.

   _____

340. Peripheral neuropathy in patients with HIV-1 infection can be caused by treatment with anti-retroviral agents.

   _____

341. Risk factors for burns in adults include each of the following *except:*

   a. Alcoholism
   b. Anxiety disorders
   c. Drug abuse
   d. Dementia
   e. Depression

   _____

342. Risk factors for burns in children and adolescents include each of the following *except*:

   a. School phobia
   b. Poverty
   c. Neglect
   d. Learning disabilities
   e. Family discord

   _____

*Questions 343-348 are **true-false** questions.*

343. More than 50% of individuals develop major depression in the first 6 months following spinal cord injury.

   _____

344. Reflexogenic erections status after spinal cord injury are mediated by sacral nerves and initiated by physical contact with or without erotic meaning.

   _____

345. Psychogenic erections after spinal cord injury are the result of erotic thoughts and fantasies and are mediated by sympathetic nerves.

   _____

346. Of all the attributes in physicians and nurses, the most highly valued by terminally ill patients are expertise and knowledge.

   _____

347. When the decision has been made to provide comfort measures to the terminally ill, less attention need be paid to the patient.

   _____

348. Dying persons have no more relish for somber faces than anyone else.

   _____

349. Delivery of bad news to a patient should involve each of the following *except*:

   a. A rehearsed statement that can be delivered calmly
   b. A brief statement about the news
   c. A statement that encourages further discussion
   d. A statement that assures the patient and promises continued attention and care
   e. A statement that encourages the patient to be strong for the sake of others.

   ————

*Questions 350-351 are **true-false** questions.*

350. Most studies of patients who were asked if they wanted to be told the truth about malignancy overwhelmingly indicated their desire for the truth.

   ————

351. The World Health Organization (WHO) defines palliative or hospice care as the active total care of patients who are dying.

   ————

352. In the Netherlands, the most frequent reason for a request for euthanasia is:
   a. Loss of dignity
   b. Pain
   c. Unworthy dying
   d. Being dependent on others
   e. Being tired of life

   ————

*Questions 353-356 are **true-false** questions.*

353. It is psychologically more difficult to stop a treatment (e.g., mechanical ventilation) once it has been started than to discontinue one.

   ————

354. Competent patients with a reversible illness have the right to refuse treatment, including life-saving treatment.

   ————

355. In a persistent vegetative state, when the patient has a functioning brain stem, but a total loss of cortical function, the eyes may open spontaneously but do not track.

   ————

356. When the patient is irreversibly ill and dying, cardiopulmonary resuscitation (CPR) is not a medical option.

   ————

357. Psychiatric units in general hospitals were first opened:

   a. Between 1900 and 1910
   b. Between 1910 and 1920
   c. Between 1930 and 1940
   d. Between 1940 and 1950
   e. After 1950

   ————

358. Each of the following statements, regarding what the physician should do before prescribing psychotropic medication, is true *except*:

    a. It is important to establish diagnostic hypotheses.
    b. It is important to be aware of potential medical problems or drug interactions.
    c. It is important to be aware of the possibility for alcohol and substance abuse.
    d. It is important to enlist the cooperation of family and friends.
    e. It is important to identify target symptoms.

    _____

*Questions 359-362 are **true-false** questions.*

359. In general, it is wise to warn patients in advance about side effects they might experience.

    _____

360. In general, the elderly require doses of psychotropics similar to those used in middle age.

    _____

361. Physicians are restricted by the FDA from using an approved drug for a non-approved condition.

    _____

362. The cost of psychotropics is rarely important in treatment selection.

    _____

363. Antipsychotic drugs have been in clinical use since:

    a. The 1930s
    b. The 1940s
    c. The 1950s
    d. The 1960s
    e. The 1970s.

    _____

*Questions 364-366 are **true-false** questions.*

364. Typical antipsychotic drugs that produce extrapyramidal symptoms are high-affinity antagonists of D_2 dopamine receptors.

    _____

365. Clozapine has a lower propensity for causing EPS than chlorpromazine.

    _____

366. All antipsychotics available in the United States, except clozapine, are high-affinity D_2 dopamine receptor antagonists.

    _____

Questions 367-371 involve matching the drug class in the left-hand column with the drug name, to which it belongs, in the right-hand column.

367. _____Piperazine phenothiazine   a. Pimozide

368. _____Dibenzodiazepine   b. Fluphenazine

369. _____Butyrophenone   c. Thioridazine

370. _____Diphenylbutylpiperidine   d. Clozapine

371. _____Piperidine phenothiazine   e. Haloperidol

*Questions 372-374 are **true-false** questions.*

372. Piperidine-substituted phenothiazines are more anticholinergic and have a lower incidence of EPS than non-piperidine-substituted phenothiazines.

_____

373. Haloperidol is a shorter-acting butyrophenone than is droperidol.

_____

374. Pimozide's half-life is shorter than haloperidol's half-life.

_____

Questions 375-379 involve matching the drug in the left-hand column with the number of milligrams in the right-hand column, so that all drugs listed are paired as mg-equivalents.

375. _____ Chlorpromazine   a. 2 mg

376. _____ Perphenazine   b. 100 mg

377. _____ Trifluoperazine   c. 95 mg

378. _____ Loxapine   d. 1 mg

379. _____ Haloperidol   e. 5 mg

Questions 380-384 involve matching the drug in the left-hand column with the number of milligrams in the right-hand column, so that all drugs listed are paired in mg-equivalents.

380. _____Thioridazine   a. 5 mg

381. _____Fluphenazine   b. 8 mg

382. _____Thiothixene   c. 10 mg

383. _____Clozapine   d. 100 mg

384. _____Pimozide   e. 2 mg

385. Which of the following drugs has the *greatest* sedative effect?

   a. Fluphenazine
   b. Chlorpromazine
   c. Perphenazine
   d. Thiothixene
   e. Risperidone

   _____

386. Which of the following drugs has the *lowest* sedative effect?

   a. Thioridazine
   b. Risperidone
   c. Clozapine
   d. Loxapine
   e. Mesoridazine

   _____

387. Which of the following drugs *most* often has a hypotensive effect?

   a. Thiothixene
   b. Chlorpromazine
   c. Fluphenazine
   d. Trifluoperazine
   e. Haloperidol

   _____

388. Which of the following drugs *least* often has a hypotensive effect?

   a. Haloperidol
   b. Clozapine
   c. Thioridazine
   d. Chlorpromazine
   e. Loxapine

   _____

389. Which of the following drugs has the *greatest* anticholinergic effect?

   a. Chlorpromazine
   b. Thiothixene
   c. Clozapine
   d. Haloperidol
   e. Risperidone

   _____

390. Which of the following drugs has the *least* anticholinergic effect?

   a. Risperidone
   b. Clozapine
   c. Thioridazine
   d. Chlorpromazine
   e. Loxapine

   _____

391. Which of the following drugs has the **greatest** chance of causing EPS?

    a. Pimozide
    b. Risperidone
    c. Clozapine
    d. Thioridazine
    e. Chlorpromazine

    _____

392. Which of the following drugs is **least** often associated with EPS?

    a. Haloperidol
    b. Chlorpromazine
    c. Fluphenazine
    d. Trifluoperazine
    e. Molindone

    _____

Questions 393-400 are **true-false** *questions.*

393. In general, excluding risperidone, low-potency antipsychotics tend to be more sedating, more anticholinergic, and cause more postural hypotension than high-potency agents.

    _____

394. The only antipsychotic drug approved by the FDA for IV administration is droperidol.

    _____

395. Long-acting depot preparations of neuroleptics include fluphenazine decanoate and haloperidol decanoate.

    _____

396. Haloperidol decanoate has a shorter half-life than does fluphenazine decanoate.

    _____

397. Blood levels of antipsychotics correlate well with clinical response.

    _____

398. Thioridazine and pimozide are potent calcium channel blockers.

    _____

399. Most antipsychotics are potent antiemetics.

    _____

400. Antipsychotics can effectively control choreoathetotic movements of Huntington's disease.

    _____

401. Indications for the use of antipsychotic drugs include each of the following **except**:

    a. Mania
    b. Tourette's syndrome
    c. Hallucinogen-induced psychosis
    d. Huntington's disease
    e. Parkinson's disease

    _____

402. Long-term use of typical antipsychotics is associated with which of the following?

    a. Huntington's disease
    b. Tourette's syndrome
    c. Torsade de pointes
    d. Hemiballismus
    e. Tardive dyskinesia

    _____

*Questions 403-405 are **true-false** questions*

403. The FDA has limited the dosage approved for pimozide to 12 mg per day for Tourette's syndrome.

_____

404. Co-administration of benztropine (1 to 2 mg per day) along with a neuroleptic decreases the incidence of acute dystonia.

_____

405. A substantial number of schizophrenic patients fail to benefit from standard antipsychotic drugs.

_____

406. Fluphenazine decanoate 0.5 ml every 2 weeks is roughly equivalent to how many mg per day of fluphenazine hydrochloride?

a. 2
b. 5
c. 10
d. 15
e. 25

_____

407. The ratio of haloperidol decanoate to oral haloperidol is approximately:

a. 1 to 1
b. 2 to 1
c. 5-10 to 1
d. 10-15 to 1
e. 20 to 1

_____

*Questions 408-409 are **true-false** questions.*

408. Haloperidol decanoate 150 mg given every 4 weeks is roughly equivalent to 30 mg per day of oral haloperidol.

_____

409. Clozapine has not been found helpful in L-dopa–induced psychotic symptoms.

_____

410. The rate of clozapine-induced agranulocytosis is approximately:

a. 1%
b. 2%
c. 3%
d. 5%
e. 7%

_____

*Questions 411-412 are **true-false** questions.*

411. Greater than 95% of cases of agranulocytosis occur within the first 2 months of treatment with clozapine.

_____

412. Most clozapine-responsive patients are effectively treated with doses of 200 to 300 mg per day.

_____

413. At doses greater than 600 mg per day of clozapine, the risk of seizures increases to:

    a. 1%-2%
    b. 3%-5%
    c. 6%-8%
    d. 9%-11%
    e. Greater than 12%

    ———

414. Side effects of clozapine include each of the following *except*:

    a. Tachycardia
    b. Weight gain
    c. Sedation
    d. Hypertension
    e. Hypersalivation

    ———

415. *True-false*. Risperidone has a high affinity for the 5-HT$_2$ receptor.

    ———

416. Each of the following statements about acute dystonias associated with neuroleptic medication is true *except*:

    a. It is likely to occur in the first week of treatment.
    b. It has a higher incidence in patients less than 40 years old.
    c. It can be treated with parenteral benztropine or diphenhydramine.
    d. It has a higher incidence in males.
    e. It is more common with low potency agents.

    ———

417. Commonly used anti-parkinsonism drugs include each of the following *except*:

    a. Benztropine
    b. Biperiden
    c. Trihexyphenidyl
    d. Amantadine
    e. Bromocriptine

    ———

418. Symptoms of antipsychotic-induced parkinsonism include each of the following *except*:

    a. Cog-wheeling
    b. Tremor
    c. Drooling
    d. Myoclonus
    e. Festination

    ———

419. *True-false*. Neuroleptic malignant syndrome (NMS) is a dose-related neuroleptic-induced syndrome.

    ———

420. Symptoms associated with NMS include each of the following *except*:

    a. Fever
    b. Rigidity
    c. Miosis
    d. Tachycardia
    e. Autonomic instability

    ———

421. Treatment of NMS includes each of the following *except*:

    a. Adequate hydration
    b. Dantrolene
    c. Bromocriptine
    d. Benztropine
    e. Amantadine

    ———

*Questions 422-424 are **true-false** questions.*

422. Dantrolene is a direct-acting muscle relaxant, which may decrease rigidity, secondary hyperthermia, and tachycardia associated with NMS.

_____

423. At least one-third of patients treated with neuroleptics over a period of years will develop tardive dyskinesia.

_____

424. Tardive dyskinesia rarely develops within 6 months of initiation of neuroleptic treatment.

_____

425. Pigmentary retinopathy is most closely associated with the use of high doses of which of the following neuroleptics?

a. Thioridazine
b. Chlorpromazine
c. Haloperidol
d. Thiothixene
e. Perphenazine

_____

426. A major endocrinological impact of typical antipsychotics is:

a. Hypothyroidism
b. Hyperparathyroidism
c. Hyperprolactinemia
d. SIADH
e. Hypercalcemia

_____

*Questions 427-428 are **true-false** questions.*

427. The most common reasons for failure of an antidepressant drug trial used for the treatment of depression are inadequate drug dosage and inadequate length of drug trial.

_____

428. Fewer than 25% of bipolar patients develop a manic episode during treatment with an antidepressant drug.

_____

429. Patients with atypical depression report each of the following symptoms *except*:

a. Rejection sensitivity
b. Insomnia
c. Mood reactivity
d. Hyperphagia
e. Fatigue

_____

430. Which of the following antidepressants has been linked to tardive dyskinesia after long-term use?

a. Phenelzine
b. Desipramine
c. Amitriptyline
d. Fluoxetine
e. Amoxapine

_____

431. Which of the following descriptions of an EEG is **most** likely to be seen in cases of benzodiazepine intoxication?

    a. Increased beta activity
    b. Theta activity
    c. Fronto-central spike and wave
    d. Generalized 3-Hz spike and wave
    e. Periodic lateralizing epileptiform discharges

    ———

432. Which of the following agents has significant anti-obsessional activity?

    a. Protriptyline
    b. Desipramine
    c. Nortriptyline
    d. Clomipramine
    e. Doxepin

    ———

433. Which of the following agents has been associated with seizures in a study of bulimics?

    a. Amoxapine
    b. Bupropion
    c. Clomipramine
    d. Desipramine
    e. Nortriptyline

    ———

434. **True-false**. Roughly the same serum levels of amitriptyline need to be achieved for the treatment of neuropathic pain as for depression.

    ———

Questions 435-439 involve matching the drug name in the left-hand column with the usual daily dosage, in milligrams per day, in the right-hand column.

435. _____ Fluoxetine   a. 75-100

436. _____ Sertraline   b. 15-40

437. _____ Nortriptyline   c. 20

438. _____ Protriptyline   d. 100-150

439. _____ Clomipramine   e. 150-200

440. **True-false**. The therapeutic plasma level of nortriptyline is 150-250 ng/ml.

    ———

Questions 441-445 involve matching the drug name in the left-hand column with the usual daily dosage, in milligrams per day, in the right-hand column.

441. _____Phenelzine   a. 200-300

442. _____Tranylcypromine   b. 75-225

443. _____Bupropion   c. 30-50

444. _____Venlafaxine   d. 20

445. _____Paroxetine   e. 45-60

446. Which of the following agents is the ***most*** sedating?

    a. Clomipramine
    b. Imipramine
    c. Nortriptyline
    d. Paroxetine
    e. Bupropion

_____

447. Which of the following agents is the ***most*** sedating?

    a. Amoxapine
    b. Doxepin
    c. Desipramine
    d. Protriptyline
    e. Phenelzine

_____

448. Which of the following agents is the ***least*** sedating?

    a. Trazodone
    b. Trimipramine
    c. Tranylcypromine
    d. Maprotiline
    e. Amitriptyline

_____

449. Which of the following agents is the ***least*** sedating?

    a. Maprotiline
    b. Doxepin
    c. Imipramine
    d. Venlafaxine
    e. Trimipramine

_____

450. Which of the following agents is the ***most*** anticholinergic?

    a. Amoxapine
    b. Desipramine
    c. Nortriptyline
    d. Maprotiline
    e. Clomipramine

_____

451. Which of the following agents is the ***most*** anticholinergic?

    a. Fluoxetine
    b. Venlafaxine
    c. Trazodone
    d. Doxepin
    e. Phenelzine

_____

452. Which of the following agents is the *least* anticholinergic?

    a. Nefazodone
    b. Amitriptyline
    c. Doxepin
    d. Protriptyline
    e. Amoxapine

    ———

453. Which of the following agents is the *least* anticholinergic?

    a. Clomipramine
    b. Bupropion
    c. Imipramine
    d. Nortriptyline
    e. Amoxapine

    ———

454. Which of the following agents is the *most* likely to cause orthostatic hypotension?

    a. Clomipramine
    b. Nortriptyline
    c. Protriptyline
    d. Paroxetine
    e. Bupropion

    ———

455. Which of the following agents is the *most* likely to cause orthostatic hypotension?

    a. Nortriptyline
    b. Imipramine
    c. Protriptyline
    d. Paroxetine
    e. Sertraline

    ———

456. SSRI-induced sexual dysfunction may be effectively treated by use of each of the following *except*:

    a. Cyproheptadine
    b. Bupropion
    c. Imipramine
    d. Yohimbine
    e. Amantadine

    ———

*Questions 457-460 are **true-false** questions.*

457. Paroxetine is the SSRI with the most potent inhibition of the P450 2D6 cytochrome system.

    ———

458. The half-life of fluoxetine is at least twice as long as is sertraline's half-life.

    ———

459. Fluvoxamine's only FDA-approved indication is for treatment of OCD.

    ———

460. Lithium treatment can be augmented by use of L-triiodothyronine in doses of 25-50 mg per day.

    ———

461. Priapism, although rare with use of antidepressants, is thought to be *most* likely with which of the following agents?

    a. Bupropion
    b. Desipramine
    c. Nortriptyline
    d. Trazodone
    e. Venlafaxine

    ———

462. Neuropsychological testing is often used as an adjunct to the assessment of each of the following *except:*

    a. Debilitation
    b. Dementia
    c. Depression
    d. Neurological disease
    e. Neurosurgical interventions

    ———

463. Iproniazid, the first of the MAOIs, was synthesized and used in the 1950s to treat which of the following conditions?

    a. Anemia
    b. Hepatitis
    c. Hypertension
    d. Syphilis
    e. Tuberculosis

    ———

464. *True-false.* For phenelzine, inhibition of greater than 85% of MAOI-type B activity appears to correlate with therapeutic efficacy.

    ———

465. The therapeutic value of lithium, as a mood stabilizer, was noted serendipitously in 1949 by:

    a. Schou
    b. Cade
    c. Kety
    d. Jefferson
    e. Yassa

    ———

466. Lithium was first approved by the FDA for the treatment of mania in what year?

    a. 1950
    b. 1955
    c. 1960
    d. 1965
    e. 1970

    ———

467. Each of the following statements about lithium is true *except:*

    a. Lithium levels are based on measurements 10-12 hours after the last dose.
    b. Lithium circulates unbound to plasma proteins.
    c. Lithium levels are decreased by thiazides by 30% to 50%.
    d. Lithium has a smaller volume of distribution in the elderly.
    e. Lithium is excreted almost entirely by the kidney.

    ———

*Questions 468-469 are **true-false** questions.*

468. Lithium inhibits the coupling of certain neurotransmitter receptors to G proteins and to second messenger systems.

    ———

469. Lithium is effective treatment for manic episodes in approximately 55% to 65% of cases.

    ———

470. Lithium use is associated with each of the following *except*:

   a. Sino-atrial node dysfunction
   b. Elevation of the white blood cell count
   c. Hypothyroidism
   d. Hyperprolactinemia
   e. Tremor

   _____

*Questions 471-472 are **true-false** questions.*

471. When a bipolar patient is recovering from surgery on the gastrointestinal tract, lithium may be administered parenterally.

   _____

472. Severe neurotoxicity is almost always present when lithium levels rise above 3.0 mmol per liter.

   _____

473. Amiloride is often used in which of the following conditions?

   a. Lithium-induced nephrotic syndrome
   b. Lithium-induced polyuria
   c. Acute renal failure
   d. Interstitial nephritis
   e. Glomerulosclerosis

   _____

474. Overall, what percent of patients receiving long-term lithium therapy develop hypothyroidism?

   a. 1
   b. 3
   c. 5
   d. 10
   e. 20

   _____

475. Roughly what percent of lithium-treated patients will develop a goiter?

   a. 1
   b. 3
   c. 5
   d. 10
   e. 20

   _____

476. Which of the following is the most common dermatological reaction associated with lithium treatment?

   a. Acne
   b. Hair loss
   c. Psoriasis
   d. Rash
   e. Folliculitis

   _____

477. Agents known to raise lithium levels include each of the following *except*:

   a. Thiazide diuretics
   b. Nonsteroidal antiinflammatory drugs
   c. Theophylline
   d. ACE inhibitors
   e. Tetracycline

   _____

478. Valproic acid is **least** effective for which of the following disorders?

   a. Absence seizures
   b. Myoclonic seizures
   c. Generalized seizures
   d. Partial seizures
   e. Bipolar disorder

   _____

Questions 479-482 are true-false questions.

479. Divalproex sodium is an enteric-coated form that contains equal parts of valproic acid and sodium valproate.

_____

480. Divalproex sodium is more slowly absorbed than is valproic acid.

_____

481. Valproic acid's half-life is 16-20 hours.

_____

482. Valproic acid's mechanism of action is the inhibition of GABA.

_____

483. Carbamazepine is *least* effective in which of the following conditions?

a. Trigeminal neuralgia
b. Complex partial seizures
c. PTSD
d. Generalized seizures
e. Neuropathic pain

_____

484. *True/false.* Therapeutic levels of carbamazepine are in the range of 4-12 mcg/ml for epilepsy and 8-12 mcg/ml for bipolar disorder.

_____

485. Clonazepam is *least* effective in which of the following conditions?

a. Petit mal seizures
b. Complex partial seizures
c. Myoclonic seizures
d. Schizoaffective disorder
e. Panic disorder

_____

486. Neuropsychological testing can be complicated or impractical in each of the following *except:*

a. The aphasic patient
b. The aprosodic patient
c. The intubated patient
d. The quadriplegic patient
b. The visually impaired patient

_____

487. Levels of carbamazepine are increased by use of each of the following *except*:

a. Cimetidine
b. SSRIs
c. Isoniazid
d. Phenytoin
e. Erythromycin

_____

488. Which of the following is a rare, potentially fatal syndrome associated with carbamazepine treatment?

a. Serotonin syndrome
b. Catatonia
c. NMS
d. Malignant hyperthermia
e. Stevens-Johnson syndrome

_____

489. The state in which the cessation of long-term use of benzodiazepines results in pathologic signs and symptoms is known as which of the following?

    a. Addiction
    b. Dependence
    c. Tolerance
    d. Habituation
    e. Intoxication

    _____

490. Withdrawal symptoms from benzodiazepine-cessation include each of the following *except*:

    a. Tachycardia
    b. Hyperreflexia
    c. Hypertension
    d. Constipation
    e. Tremulousness

    _____

*Questions 491-492 are **true-false** questions.*

491. All highly addicting drugs produce a physiological withdrawal syndrome.

    _____

492. Antacids interfere with absorption of benzodiazepines from the GI tract.

    _____

Questions 493-497 involve matching the drug in the left-hand column with the number of milligrams in the right-hand column so that each agent is matched with its milligram equivalent dosage.

493. _____ Alprazolam   a. 0.25

494. _____ Chlordiazepoxide   b. 7.5

495. _____ Clonazepam   c. 0.5

496. _____ Clorazepate   d. 5

497. _____ Diazepam   e. 10

Questions 498-502 involve matching the drug in the left-hand column with the number of milligrams in the right-hand column so that each agent is matched with its milligram equivalent dosage.

498. _____ Estazolam   a. 1

499. _____ Flurazepam   b. 15

500. _____ Lorazepam   c. 30

501. _____ Oxazepam   d. 2

502. _____ Triazolam   e. 0.25

Questions 503-507 involve matching the drug in the left-hand column with the half-life listed for that drug in the right-hand column.

503. _____ Alprazolam   a. 30-100

504. _____ Clonazepam   b. 6-20

505. _____ Clorazepate   c. 1.5-5

506. _____ Flurazepam   d. 18-50

507. _____ Triazolam   e. 50-160

*Questions 508-515 are **true-false** questions.*

508. Clorazepate has a more rapid onset of action than does alprazolam.

_____

509. Lorazepam, oxazepam, and triazolam are metabolized only by conjugation with glucuronic acid; no intermediate steps and no active metabolites are present.

_____

510. Benzodiazepines and barbiturates act at separate binding sites on the $GABA_A$ receptor to potentiate the inhibiting action of GABA. They do so by allosterically regulating the receptor so that it has a greater infinity for GABA.

_____

511. Zolpidem, used for the short-term treatment of insomnia, lacks significant muscle relaxant and anticonvulsant effects.

_____

512. Buspirone is a non-benzodiazepine anxiolytic with no direct effect on $GABA_A$ receptors.

_____

513. Buspirone is believed to exert its anxiolytic effect as a partial antagonist of $5\text{-}HT_{1A}$ receptors.

_____

514. Although buspirone is completely absorbed in the GI tract, it undergoes extensive first-pass metabolism in the liver.

_____

515. Buspirone, though not a benzodiazepine, cross-reacts with benzodiazepines and can be used to prevent benzodiazepine withdrawal syndromes.

_____

516. Benzodiazepines affect sleep architecture in several ways. Each of the following is true about benzodiazepines *except*:

    a. Benzodiazepines suppress REM sleep
    b. Benzodiazepines shorten REM latency
    c. Benzodiazepines increase stage 2 sleep
    d. Benzodiazepines decrease stages 1, 3, and 4 sleep
    e. Benzodiazepines reduce sleep fragmentation.

    _____

517. *True-false*. Parenteral lorazepam can reverse both neuroleptic-induced and psychogenic catatonia.

    _____

518. Each of the following agents increases the levels of benzodiazepines that are demethylated and hydroxylated *except*:

    a. Cimetidine
    b. Carbamazepine
    c. Disulfiram
    d. Erythromycin
    e. SSRIs

    _____

519. The Wisconsin Card Sorting Test is primarily used for the assessment of:

    a. Cerebellar function
    b. Frontal lobe function
    c. Occipital lobe function
    d. Parietal lobe function
    e. Temporal lobe function

    _____

*Questions 520-524 are **true-false** questions.*

520. At the present time, psychostimulants are classified as schedule III drugs.

    _____

521. Psychostimulants, while approved by the FDA only for the treatment of ADHD and narcolepsy, are also used to potentiate the effects of narcotic analgesics.

    _____

522. The half-life of dextroamphetamine is shorter than the half-life of methylphenidate.

    _____

523. Pemoline's half-life enables once daily dosing, but its therapeutic actions in ADHD are usually delayed by 3-4 weeks.

    _____

524. Chronic use of high-dose amphetamine may produce stereotypic movements.

    _____

525. Each of the following statements about narcolepsy is true *except*:

    a. It is a disorder of excessive daytime sleepiness
    b. It is manifest by irresistible sleep attacks of short duration
    c. It is associated with cataplexy, which is often preceded by strong emotions
    d. It is associated with anger attacks
    e. It is associated with hypnagogic hallucinations.

    _____

526. High doses of psychostimulants may result in each of the following *except*:

    a. Bruxism
    b. Formication
    c. Irritability
    d. Paranoia
    e. Miosis

    _____

*Questions 527-532 are **true-false** questions.*

527. β-Adrenergic receptor antagonists are effective in the treatment of performance anxiety, lithium-induced tremor, and neuroleptic-induced akathisia.

    _____

528. α-1 Receptors are located postsynaptically in both the sympathetic nervous system and the brain.

    _____

529. In the brain, α-1 receptors are found on both neurons and blood vessels.

    _____

530. Stimulation of α-1 receptors causes vasodilatation.

    _____

531. For patients with asthma or other obstructive pulmonary disorders, a relatively selective β-1 antagonist, like atenolol, is preferred.

    _____

532. Clonidine's principal mechanism of action appears to be as an α-2 adrenergic receptor antagonist in the CNS.

    _____

533. Clonidine is used for each of the following *except*:

    a. Opioid withdrawal
    b. Tourette's syndrome
    c. Hypertension
    d. Sleep apnea
    e. Neuroleptic-induced akathisia

    _____

534. Each of the following drugs increases the severity of disulfiram-alcohol reactions **except**:

    a. MAOIs
    b. Vasopressors
    c. TCAs
    d. Neuroleptics
    e. α-Adrenergic antagonists

    _____

*Questions 535-537 are **true-false** questions.*

535. Tacrine is a reversible inhibitor of acetylcholine.

    _____

536. By inhibiting the metabolism of acetylcholine in the brain, tacrine is thought to ameliorate the partial depletion of this neurotransmitter brought about by the drop out of cholinergic neurons.

    _____

537. Approximately 10% of patients on tacrine develop elevations in hepatic amino transferase activity.

_____

538. Which of the following is *not* a feature of anticholinergic delirium?

   a. A positive response to IV physostigmine
   b. Tachycardia
   c. Fever
   d. Diaphoresis
   e. Mydriasis

_____

539. Which of the following is *not* a feature of serotonin syndrome?

   a. Muscle rigidity
   b. Diaphoresis
   c. Autonomic instability
   d. Tremor
   e. Hyperreflexia

_____

540. Which of the following is *not* used in the treatment of NMS?

   a. Amantadine
   b. Bromocriptine
   c. Dantrolene
   d. Hydroxyzine
   e. Nondepolarizing paralytic agents

_____

541. Catatonia is *most* often seen in association with which of the following conditions?

   a. Affective illness
   b. Hypercalcemia
   c. Conversion disorder
   d. Parkinson's disease
   e. Schizophrenia

_____

542. Which of the following is *not* associated with the successful treatment of catatonia?

   a. ECT
   b. IV amobarbital
   c. IV lorazepam
   d. IV dantrolene
   e. Neuroleptic administration

_____

543. Catatonia was first described by which of the following physicians?

   a. Eugen Bleuler
   b. Alan Gelenberg
   c. Karl Kahlbaum
   d. Seymour Kety
   e. Emil Kraepelin

_____

544. Which of the following medical conditions, detected during an examination of a patient, does *not* heighten the probability that an alcohol use disorder is present?

   a. Pancreatitis
   b. Gastrointestinal bleeding
   c. Sleep disorder
   d. Cataracts
   e. Cardiomyopathy

_____

545. Which of the following is *not* typically associated with alcohol intoxication?

   a. Ataxia
   b. Delirium
   c. Disinhibition
   d. Dysarthria
   e. Hypoglycemia

_____

546. Which of the following benzodiazepines is often recommended for detoxification of the alcohol-dependent individual with hepatitis?

    a. Alprazolam
    b. Chlordiazepoxide
    c. Clonazepam
    d. Clorazepate
    e. Lorazepam

    _____

547. Which of the following is an opiate antagonist that has recently been found to reduce craving and relapse in alcoholics?

    a. Disulfiram
    b. Flumazenil
    c. Naloxone
    d. Natrexone
    e. Phentolamine

    _____

548. Which of the following statements about disulfiram is *false*?

    a. It inhibits dopamine β-hydroxylase.
    b. It may induce pancreatitis.
    c. It may elevate levels of acetaldehyde.
    d. It can produce tachycardia, dyspnea, and vomiting if alcohol is ingested.
    e. It can exacerbate psychosis in some schizophrenics.

    _____

549. Which of the following complications is *least* often associated with cocaine abuse and dependence?

    a. Abruptio placentae
    b. Generalized seizures
    c. Sexual dysfunction
    d. Pulmonary hypertension
    e. Cardiac arrhythmias

    _____

550. Which of the following features is *not* associated with opiate withdrawal?

    a. Diaphoresis
    b. Lacrimation
    c. Miotic pupils
    d. Rhinorrhea
    e. Yawning

    _____

551. Which of the following orally administered medications is *not* roughly equivalent to a 5-mg oral dose of diazepam?

    a. Alprazolam 0.5 mg
    b. Clorazepate 7.5 mg
    c. Lorazepam 1.0 mg
    d. Midazolam 5 mg
    e. Chlordiazepoxide 10 mg

    _____

552. Which of the following benzodiazepines has the *shortest* half-life?

    a. Oxazepam
    b. Clorazepate
    c. Diazepam
    d. Chlordiazepoxide
    e. Clonazepam

    _____

553. Which of the following TCAs is *least* likely to induce orthostatic hypotension?

    a. Amitriptyline
    b. Doxepin
    c. Desipramine
    d. Imipramine
    e. Nortriptyline

    _____

554. TCA-induced orthostatic hypotension is *least* likely to be associated with which of the following?

a. Congestive heart failure
b. Advanced age
c. Pre-drug orthostatic fall in blood pressure
d. Anticholinergic potency
e. Bundle branch block

_____

555. Which of the following electrocardiographic findings is *not* commonly associated with TCA use?

a. Prolongation of QRS segment
b. Prolongation of QTc
c. Prolongation of PR interval
d. Development of flattened T-waves
e. Development of U-waves

_____

556. Which of the following is *not* true about MAOI therapy?

a. MAOI use can lead to hypertensive crises.
b. MAOI-induced orthostatic hypotension can be treated with fludrocortisone.
c. MAOI-induced orthostatic hypotension can be predicted by pre-MAOI orthostatic falls in blood pressure.
d. MAOI-induced hypotension can be treated with 1-inch cubes of cheddar cheese.
e. MAOI-induced hypotension is often worse after the 3rd or 4th week.

_____

557. Thioridazine has roughly the same anticholinergic potency as which of the following agents?

a. Bupropion
b. Trazodone
c. Desipramine
d. Protriptyline
e. Fluoxetine

_____

558. Lithium therapy is *least* likely to be associated with which of the following electrocardiographic findings?

a. Sinus node dysfunction
b. T-wave flattening
c. QRS prolongation
d. T-wave inversion
e. First-degree block

_____

559. In a depressed patient with untreated atrial fibrillation, which of the following classes of antidepressants at usual dosages would be most likely to result in a rapid ventricular response?

a. MAOIs
b. Lithium
c. TCAs
d. SSRIs
e. Psychostimulants

_____

560. TCAs are *least* likely to be associated with which of the following?

    a. The development of Ebstein's anomaly
    b. Impaired conduction in the H-V portion of a His bundle
    c. Orthostatic hypotension that precedes therapeutic effects
    d. Sudden death if the QTc exceeds 440 milliseconds
    e. Proarrhythmic effects following myocardial infarction

    _____

561. What is the recommended upper limit dose of a TCA for children?

    a. 1 mg/kg/d
    b. 3 mg/kg/d
    c. 5 mg/kg/d
    d. 7 mg/kg/d
    e. 9 mg/kg/d

    _____

562. Of the agents listed below, which is associated with the *greatest* effects on cardiac conduction?

    a. Alprazolam
    b. Bupropion
    c. Sertraline
    d. Thioridazine
    e. Tranylcypromine

    _____

563. The patient whose condition is delineated by the voluntary production of symptoms, presumably in order to assume the patient role, likely has which of the following conditions?

    a. Hypochondriasis
    b. Malingering
    c. Factitious disorder
    d. Conversion disorder
    e. Somatization disorder

    _____

564. The patient who voluntarily produces signs and symptoms as a means of achieving clear-cut secondary gain likely has which of the following conditions?

    a. Hypochondriasis
    b. Malingering
    c. Factitious disorder
    d. Conversion disorder
    e. Somatization disorder

    _____

565. The name for the Münchausen's syndrome was coined in 1951 by which of the following?

    a. Howard Spiro
    b. Richard Asher
    c. Marvin Stern
    d. Charles Ford
    e. Karl Friedrich Heironymus von Münchausen

    _____

566. Which is *not* an alternative label for a patient with Münchausen syndrome?

    a. Hospital hobo
    b. Peregrinating problem patient
    c. Sufferer of Ahasuerus syndrome
    d. Hospital addict
    e. Somatizer

    _____

567. Which of the following features is *not* characteristic of Münchausen syndrome?

    a. An evasive manner
    b. A multiplicity of scars
    c. A labile affect
    d. An acute, but not entirely convincing, history
    e. Numerous forms of identification

    _____

568. Which of the following is **not** associated with a well-known variety of factitious illness?

    a. The self-administration of anticoagulants
    b. The administration of laxatives to a child
    c. The creation of self-inflicted wounds
    d. The self-injection of foreign bodies into body parts
    e. The belief that one is ill despite extensive work-ups

    ———

569. Which of the following terms is used to describe a chronic syndrome beginning by age 30 with multiple symptoms that are unexplained by medical work-ups and with psychosocial distress?

    a. Hypochondriasis
    b. Conversion disorder
    c. Somatization disorder
    d. Factitious illness
    e. Malingering

    ———

570. Which of the following conditions is **least** likely to be confused with somatization disorder?

    a. Acute intermittent porphyria
    b. Systemic lupus erythematosus
    c. Multiple sclerosis
    d. Acute Guillain-Barré syndrome
    e. Brucellosis

    ———

571. Which of the following conditions involves a loss or change in bodily functions that results from a psychological conflict or need?

    a. Hypochondriasis
    b. Conversion disorder
    c. Somatization disorder
    d. Factitious disorder
    e. Malingering

    ———

572. Which of the following conditions is associated with preoccupation with bodily health and physiologic functioning, elaborate self-treatment, and frequent visits with physicians?

    a. Hypochondriasis
    b. Conversion disorder
    c. Somatization disorder
    d. Factitious disorder
    e. Malingering

    ———

573. Which of the following conditions may involve somatic delusions?

    a. Organic brain syndrome
    b. Panic disorder
    c. Obsessive-compulsive disorder
    d. Hypochondriasis
    e. Somatization disorder

    ———

574. Which of the following conditions is associated with a decreased sensitivity to opiates?

    a. Hepatic impairment
    b. Head trauma
    c. Cor pulmonale
    d. Deafferentation pain
    e. Hypovolemia

    ———

575. Which of the following drugs is *not* recommended for the treatment of continuous pain in the terminally ill?

    a. Acetaminophen for mild pain
    b. Codeine and nonsteroidal antiinflammatory drugs for moderate pain
    c. Morphine for severe pain
    d. Meperidine for severe pain
    e. Steroids for bone pain

    ———

576. Which of the following is the *most* reasonable goal of chronic pain treatment?

    a. Reduction in the number of office visits
    b. Complete pain relief
    c. Restoration of function
    d. Certification of disability
    e. Treatment of depression

    ———

577. What is the percentage of cancer patients who die without experiencing pain?

    a. 3%
    b. 23%
    c. 33%
    d. 53%
    e. 73%

    ———

578. What percentage of patients with chronic pain have centrally-mediated pain?

    a. 10%
    b. 25%
    c. 50%
    d. 75%
    e. 95%

    ———

579. Which of the following categories does *not* need to be considered when assessing competency?

    a. How the patient communicates choices
    b. How the patient understands relevant information
    c. How the patient appreciates the situation and its consequences
    d. What the prevailing standards are in dominant culture
    e. Whether the patient can manipulate information rationally

    ———

580. Which of the following conditions is **most** often associated with requests for evaluation for competency?

    a. Adjustment disorder
    b. Schizophrenia
    c. Depression
    d. Organic mental disorder
    e. Mania

    ———

581. The decision as to whether a patient is competent or not is made by which of the following?

    a. Resident physician
    b. Attending physician
    c. Psychiatrist
    d. Judge
    e. Family member

    ———

582. What is the prevalence of depressive disorders during pregnancy?

    a. 2%
    b. 5%
    c. 10%
    d. 15%
    e. 20%

    ———

583. Which of the following drugs is associated with the **lowest** risk of organic dysgenesis following prenatal exposure?

a. Valproic acid
b. Lithium
c. Fluoxetine
d. Thiothixene
e. Carbamazepine

—————

584. Which of the following medications is most often associated with neural tube defects occurring after first trimester exposure?

a. Valproic acid
b. Lithium
c. Fluoxetine
d. Thiothixene
e. Desipramine

—————

585. Which of the following is **not** true about postpartum blues?

a. It occurs in approximately 5% to 10% of postpartum women.
b. It is considered a normal reaction following childbirth.
c. Its symptoms develop within 2 to 3 days of delivery.
d. Its symptoms include mood lability, tearfulness, and irritability.
e. It is a time-limited condition.

—————

586. Which of the following statements is **not** true about post-partum psychosis?

a. It is acute in onset.
b. It occurs in one to two of every 1000 postpartum women.
c. It usually leads to a diagnosis of schizophrenia.
d. It can be associated with disorganized behavior.
e. It is associated with prior postpartum psychosis.

—————

587. Postpartum depression is **not** associated with which of the following?

a. A family history of mood disorders
b. Psychosocial distress
c. Sensitivity to shifts in hormonal milieu
d. Postpartum thyroiditis
e. A prevalence of greater than 15%

—————

*Questions 588-590 are **true-false** questions.*

588. Infertility affects roughly 25% of women between 35 and 40 years of age.

—————

589. Infertility affects roughly 10% of women under 25 years of age.

—————

590. Infertility is defined as the failure to conceive after 6 months of regular sexual intercourse or the inability to carry a pregnancy to live birth.

—————

591. Which of the following statements about hyperemesis gravidarum (HG) is *true*?

    a. HG generally has its onset between 2 and 4 weeks after conception.
    b. HG generally resolves by the 16th week of pregnancy.
    c. HG develops in approximately 10 to 20 per 1000 pregnancies.
    d. HG tends to be associated with multiple gestations.
    e. HG tends to occur in underweight individuals.

    _____

592. Which of the following is *not* a complication of hyperemesis gravidarum?

    a. Hepatic dysfunction
    b. Peripheral neuropathy
    c. Renal failure
    d. Hair loss
    e. Retinal hemorrhage

    _____

593. Which of the following classes of medications is *least* likely to be effective in the treatment of HG?

    a. Antihistamines
    b. Benzodiazepines
    c. Corticosteroids
    d. Dopamine antagonists
    e. Serotonin reuptake inhibitors

    _____

594. Which of the following statements about parasomnias is *false*?

    a. They tend to occur early in the night.
    b. They are more common in children than in adults.
    c. They typically respond to treatment with carbamazepine.
    d. Individuals with parasomnias are difficult to arouse during an episode.
    e. Individuals with parasomnias may have more than one type of parasomnia.

    _____

595. Which of the following is the stage of sleep associated with sleep spindles and K complexes?

    a. Stage 1
    b. Stage 2
    c. Stage 3
    d. Stage 4
    e. REM sleep

    _____

596. REM sleep is associated with each of the following *except*:

    a. Increased muscle tone
    b. Increased penile turgidity
    c. Increased cerebral blood flow
    d. Increased oxygen consumption
    e. Increased incidence of sequential dream recall if awakened during this phase.

    _____

597. Sleep studies in the elderly typically reveal each of the following *except*:

    a. An increased number of awakenings after sleep onset
    b. An increase in daytime sleepiness
    c. A longer adjustment time to sleep-wake schedule changes
    d. An increase in sleep efficiency
    e. A reduction in the amount of NREM (delta) sleep

    _____

598. Narcolepsy is associated with each of the following *except*:

    a. Cataplexy
    b. Sleep attacks
    c. Sleep paralysis
    d. Hypnagogic hallucinations
    e. Immediate NREM sleep

    _____

599. Which of the following conditions is *least* likely to be responsible for the development of secondary mania?

    a. AIDS
    b. Multiple sclerosis
    c. Tertiary syphilis
    d. Amyotrophic lateral sclerosis
    e. Right hemisphere lesions

    _____

600. Which of the following conditions is *most* likely to be associated with symptoms of depression?

    a. Hypercalcemia
    b. Hypocalcemia
    c. Hyperkalemia
    d. Hypomagnesemia
    e. Hypertension

    _____

601. A psychiatric disorder is an *unlikely* consequence of which of the following disorders?

    a. Parkinson's disease
    b. Multiple sclerosis
    c. Amyotrophic lateral sclerosis
    d. Huntington's disease
    e. Stroke of the left frontal area

    _____

602. The *least* likely cause of a 72-year-old man's confusion and agitation two days following a motor vehicle accident (in which he sustained a brief loss of consciousness and a femur fracture) would be which of the following conditions?

    a. A subdural hematoma
    b. An epidural hematoma
    c. Fat emboli
    d. Vascular dementia
    e. Use of narcotics for pain relief

    _____

603. Cerebral emboli most often lead to infarcts supplied by which of the following arteries?

    a. Basilar artery
    b. Anterior cerebral artery
    c. Middle cerebral artery
    d. Posterior cerebral artery
    e. Vertebral artery

    _____

604. Which of the following conditions is *not* a risk factor for cerebral emboli?

    a. Atrial fibrillation
    b. Atrial flutter
    c. A patent foramen ovale
    d. Left ventricular hypokinesis
    e. Antiphospholipid antibody syndrome

    _____

605. The side-effect least commonly associated with use of selective serotonin reuptake inhibitors (SSRIs) is:

   a. Dizziness
   b. Dry mouth
   c. Erectile dysfunction
   d. Excessive sweating
   e. Nausea

606. Blockade of muscarinic receptors by tricyclic antidepressants (TCAs) is responsible for each of the following *except:*

   a. Blurred vision
   b. Constipation
   c. Orthostatic hypotension
   d. Tachycardia
   e. Urinary retention

607. Weight gain, increased appetite, and sedation are related to blockade of which type of receptors?

   a. α_1-Adrenergic receptors
   b. Cholinergic muscarinic receptors
   c. Dopamine receptors
   d. Histamine H_1 receptors
   e. None of the above

608. Which of the following is a tetracyclic antidepressant?

   a. Doxepin
   b. Escitalopram
   c. Maprotiline
   d. Nortriptyline
   e. Trimipramine

609. Which of the following antidepressants is relatively contraindicated in the treatment of patients with bulimia?

   a. Bupropion
   b. Escitalopram
   c. Mirtazapine
   d. Trazodone
   e. Venlafaxine

610. Which statement about bupropion is *false?*

   a. Blurred vision is a common side effect of bupropion.
   b. Bupropion has an extended release formulation.
   c. Bupropion is relatively contraindicated in patients with seizures.
   d. Insomnia is a common side effect of bupropion.
   e. 450 mg/day is the maximum recommended daily dose of bupropion.

611. Which type of receptor is primarily blocked by mirtazapine?

   a. α_1-Adrenergic receptors
   b. Cholinergic receptors
   c. Dopamine receptors
   d. Histaminic receptors
   e. None of the above

612. Which of the following statements about phenelzine is *false?*

a. Phenelzine inhibits both monoamine oxidase (MAO) type A and type B.
b. Phenelzine is considered to be a relatively irreversible monoamine oxidase inhibitor (MAOI).
c. Phenelzine, when combined with foods containing glutamate, can cause a hypertensive crisis.
d. Use of phenelzine is often associated with orthostatic hypotension.
e. Use of phenelzine use is often associated with weight gain.

613. Which of the following statements about electroconvulsive therapy (ECT) is *false?*

a. ECT is absolutely contraindicated in the presence of increased intracranial pressure.
b. ECT involves the application of electrical current to the skull.
c. ECT is relatively contraindicated in the presence of coronary artery disease.
d. In ECT, electrical current can be delivered by either sine-wave or brief pulse current.
e. Side effects of ECT include retrograde and anterograde amnesia.

614. Which of the following statements about antidepressants is **most** accurate?

a. Most patients show a robust response in the first month of antidepressant treatment.
b. One should only use one antidepressant at a time.
c. Phenelzine should not be started within 5 weeks of using fluoxetine.
d. TCAs uncommonly cause anticholinergic side effects.
e. Two to four weeks of antidepressant treatment is an adequate interval to determine a response.

615. Which of the following statements about suicide is *false?*

a. Anxiety disorders, especially panic disorder, are increasingly being reported among suicide victims.
b. Dependence on alcohol and other drugs is responsible for more suicides than are psychotic disorders.
c. Divorced adults are at greater risk for suicide than are those who are widowed.
d. Major depressive disorder accounts for more suicides than psychotic disorders.
e. Unemployment is associated with as many as one-half of completed suicides.

616. Which of the following statements about the evaluation of a potentially suicidal patient is *false?*

    a. A patient being evaluated for suicide must be detained until his or her risk for suicide has been assessed.
    b. Medication is indicated for the uncooperative and potentially suicidal patient.
    c. Physical restraints may be needed for patients who cannot reliably "contract" for safety.
    d. The evaluation of suicidal risk in the potentially suicidal patient takes precedence over the desire of the patient for privacy and confidentiality.
    e. The potential means for self-harm must be removed from the reach of patients at serious risk for suicide.

617. Stimulation of which of the following structures can generate panic attacks?

    a. The amygdala
    b. The anterior cingulate gyrus
    c. The left caudate nucleus
    d. The locus coeruleus
    e. The median raphe

618. Roughly what percentage of patients with atypical chest pain and normal findings on cardiac catheterization has panic disorder?

    a. <5%
    b. 5%
    c. 10%
    d. 25%
    e. 50%

619. Which of the following is *more likely* to be associated with a primary anxiety disorder than an organic anxiety syndrome?

    a. A childhood history of separation anxiety
    b. A poor response to anti-panic agents
    c. Lack of a personal or family history of an anxiety disorder
    d. Lack of avoidance behavior
    e. Onset of symptoms after the age of 35

620. Anxiety-like symptoms are associated with use of each of the following *except:*

    a. Beta-blockers
    b. Corticosteroids
    c. Sympathomimetics
    d. Theophylline
    e. Thyroid hormone

621. Medical conditions that may cause anxiety symptoms include each of the following *except:*

    a. Chronic obstructive pulmonary disease
    b. Diabetes
    c. Osteoporosis
    d. Seizure disorder
    e. Thyroid dysfunction

622. Which of the following is a syndrome characterized by discrete episodes of intense anxiety associated with at least four symptoms of autonomic arousal, and which develops rapidly and peaks within 10 minutes?

    a. Generalized anxiety disorder
    b. Panic disorder
    c. Obsessive-compulsive disorder
    d. Post-traumatic stress disorder
    e. Social phobia

    _____

623. Which of the following is a syndrome involving prior exposure to an event that involved the threat of death, injury, or harm to oneself or others?

    a. Generalized anxiety disorder
    b. Obsessive-compulsive disorder
    c. Panic disorder
    d. Post-traumatic stress disorder
    e. Social phobia

    _____

624. Which of the following statements is *true?*

    a. Midazolam is longer-lasting than diazepam.
    b. Lorazepam is less-potent than clorazepate.
    c. Oxazepam is faster-acting than clonazepam.
    d. Oxazepam is longer-lasting than clonazepam.
    e. Clorazepate is faster-acting than oxazepam.

    _____

625. Which of the following agents lacks significant metabolites?

    a. Chlordiazepoxide
    b. Clorazepate
    c. Diazepam
    d. Flurazepam
    e. Oxazepam

    _____

626. Which of the following agents has the *longest* half-life?

    a. Alprazolam
    b. Chlordiazepoxide
    c. Clorazepate
    d. Lorazepam
    e. Oxazepam

    _____

627. Which of the following is *not* usually considered a side effect of benzodiazepines?

    a. Ataxia
    b. Behavioral disinhibition
    c. Reduction in the seizure threshold
    d. Respiratory depression
    e. Sedation

    _____

628. Which of the following signs, symptoms, or manifestations is *not* generally associated with withdrawal from benzodiazepines?

    a. Constipation
    b. Insomnia
    c. Irritability
    d. Nervousness
    e. Seizures

    _____

629. Which of the following is **not** a physiological sign of acute stress?

    a. Dry mouth
    b. Fatigue
    c. Miosis
    d. Palpitations
    e. Tense muscles

    _____

630. Which of the following is **not** generally included in the evaluation of chronic stress?

    a. A determination as to whether bodily complaints follow an anatomic distribution
    b. An assessment of the individual's coping skills
    c. A search for personal social and work-related sources of stress
    d. Assessment of whether the patient's current stresses exceed their coping resources
    e. Review of the patient's insurance benefits

    _____

631. Which of the following is **not** consistent with a stress response?

    a. Current medical symptoms in the absence of a clear medical explanation
    b. Elevated digital skin temperature
    c. High electromyogram (EMG) activity of the frontalis muscle
    d. New onset of symptoms temporally related to current life stressors
    e. Tense muscles, palpitations, and diaphoresis

    _____

632. Which of the following is **not** one of the CAGE screening questions for alcohol abuse?

    a. Have people annoyed you by criticizing your drinking?
    b. Have you ever felt guilty about your drinking?
    c. Have you ever felt you should cut down on your drinking?
    d. Have you ever had a drink first thing in the morning?
    e. Have you felt it would be easy to stop drinking?

    _____

633. Which of the following statements about screening tests for alcohol abuse is **false?**

    a. Four positive responses on the CAGE test are required to diagnose significant alcohol-related problems.
    b. The Alcohol Use Disorders Identification Test (AUDIT) is a 10-item questionnaire for early detection of patients with alcohol problems in the primary care setting.
    c. The CAGE questionnaire is a 4-item screen for alcoholism.
    d. The MAST is more accurate than the CAGE for detection of alcoholism.
    e. The Michigan Alcoholism Screening Test (MAST) is a 25-item questionnaire.

    _____

634. Which of the following benzodiazepines is usually recommended for an alcohol-abusing individual (with significant liver disease) undergoing detoxification?

    a. Chlordiazepoxide
    b. Clorazepate
    c. Diazepam
    d. Flurazepam
    e. Lorazepam

_____

635. Which of the following statements about naltrexone is *false?*

    a. It is an opiate agonist.
    b. It is contraindicated in the patient with acute hepatitis.
    c. It is contraindicated in the patient with liver failure.
    d. It is often given in doses of 50 mg/day.
    e. It seems to work best in the patient who describes intense craving.

_____

636. Which of the following statements about disulfiram is *false?*

    a. Disulfiram in doses of 250 mg/day can produce tachycardia and dyspnea if the alcohol-abusing patient drinks alcohol.

    b. Disulfiram inhibits alcohol metabolism and leads to elevated levels of acetaldehyde.

    c. Disulfiram inhibits dopamine beta hydroxylase.

    d. Disulfiram is no better than placebo in producing continuous abstinence from alcohol.

    e. Use of disulfiram use does not require monitoring of liver function.

_____

637. Which of the following statements about migraine headaches is *false?*

    a. A family history of migraines is present in up to 90% of migraine sufferers.
    b. After puberty migraines are more common in women than in men.
    c. Ninety percent of migraine sufferers have their first attack by age 40.
    d. The prevalence of migraine headaches is greater in boys than in girls.
    e. The prevalence of migraines in females is approximately 5%.

_____

638. Which of the following statements about migraine headaches is *false?*

    a. A migraine headache is usually bilateral.
    b. Migraine headaches are usually severe and throbbing.
    c. Migraines are often experienced behind the eyes.
    d. Nausea and vomiting are common features of migraines.
    e. Photophobia and sonophobia are common with migraines.

_____

639. Which of the following statements about cluster headaches is **false?**

 a. Cluster headaches are the most painful type of recurrent headache.
 b. Cluster headaches come on slowly and peak in 45 -60 minutes.
 c. Injected conjunctiva, nasal blockage, and facial flushing on the side of the headache are common in cluster headache.
 d. Ptosis and miosis on the side of the pain are common with cluster headaches.
 e. Stereotyped attacks are usually present with cluster headache.

_____

640. Which of the following is **not** an acute treatment for migraines?

 a. Aspirin
 b. Fiorinal
 c. Ibuprofen
 d. Propranolol
 e. Sumatriptan

_____

641. Which of the following agents is **not** a prophylactic treatment for migraine?

 a. Phenytoin
 b. Propranolol
 c. Sodium valproate
 d. Sumatriptan
 e. Verapamil

_____

642. Which of the following is **not** a manifestation of parasomnias?

 a. Bruxism
 b. Enuresis
 c. Night terrors
 d. Restless legs
 e. Sleepwalking

_____

643. Which of the following parameters is **not** typically monitored during polysomnography?

 a. Activity of eye muscles
 b. Muscle activity
 c. Respiratory rate
 d. Skin temperature
 e. The electroencephalogram

_____

644. Which of the following is the **least** sedating?

 a. Amitriptyline
 b. Bupropion
 c. Doxepin
 d. Mirtazapine
 e. Trazodone

_____

645. Loud snoring is commonly present in patients with which of the following conditions?

 a. Chronic obstructive pulmonary disease
 b. Congestive heart failure
 c. Narcolepsy
 d. Obstructive sleep apnea
 e. Parasomnias

_____

646. Which of the following is **not** commonly associated with sleep apnea?

 a. Headache
 b. Impotence
 c. Irritability
 d. One or two episodes of apnea or hypopnea per hour of sleep
 e. Pulmonary hypertension

_____

647. Which of the following is *not* one of the classical tetrad of symptoms in narcolepsy?

    a. Cataplexy
    b. Hypnagogic hallucinations
    c. Sleep attacks
    d. Sleep paralysis
    e. Sleepwalking

———

For the following questions (648-652) match up the correct choices in each column.

648. ——— Sleepwalking

649. ——— Sleep paralysis

650. ——— Cataplexy

651. ——— Sleep attacks

652. ——— Hypnagogic hallucinations

a. Irrestible, usually brief episodes of sleep, that may occur several times each day

b. A condition involving the sudden loss of muscle tone without impaired consciousness usually triggered by emotion

c. A complete loss of muscle tone in the absence of sleep

d. A non-REM sleep state involving ambulation

e. Visual hallucinations that occur while falling asleep

For the following questions (653-657) match up the correct choices in each column.

653. ——— Bruxism

654. ——— Central sleep apne

655. ——— Night terrors

656. ——— Restless legs syndrome

657. ——— Nocturnal myoclonus

a. A condition in which no respiratory effort is made until arousal supervenes

b. A condition where achy feelings or paresthesias in the legs appear at night

c. Brief involuntary leg movements that occur every 20-40 seconds during sleep

d. A dramatic state of autonomic arousal during non-REM sleep

e. A parasomnia usually involving grinding of the teeth

658. Which of the following statements about fatigue is *false?*

    a. Fatigue is a symptom with different meanings, causes, and physical manifestations.

    b. Fatigue is an uncommon complaint in ambulatory medical settings.

    c. Fatigue is associated with high rates of anxiety and depression.

    d. Fatigue may be a normal response to exercise.

    e. Fatigue may become chronic and disabling.

————

659. Which of the following is *not* a medical cause of fatigue?

    a. Chemotherapy
    b. Hepatitis
    c. Hypothyroidism
    d. Parkinson's disease
    e. Thrombocytopenia

————

*Questions 660-664 are **true-false** questions.*

660. Anxiety disorders occur in a majority of patients with hypochondriasis.

————

661. Conversion disorder involves a change in voluntary motor or sensory function that suggests a neurological condition, but defies explanation.

————

662. The incidence of personality disorders among patients with somatoform disorders is low.

————

663. The triad of bodily preoccupation, disease fear, and disease conviction is crucial to the diagnosis of somatization disorder.

————

664. Hypochondriacal patients typically have two gastrointestinal, symptoms, one pseudoneurological symptom, four pain symptoms, and one sexual symptom.

————

665. Which of the following is *not* true regarding conversion disorder?

    a. The patient may experience a change in voluntary motor function.

    b. The patient's symptoms are a culturally sanctioned response to stress.

    c. The patient's symptoms are not intentionally produced.

    d. The patient's symptoms are presumed to be associated with psychological feelings.

    e. The symptoms may present as a single episode or as recurrent episodes.

————

666. Which of the following is **not** a criterion for somatization disorder?

    a. The patient's symptoms are intentionally feigned.
    b. The patient's symptoms begin by age 30.
    c. The symptoms are not fully explained by a known physical disorder.
    d. The symptoms cannot be caused by drugs.
    e. The symptoms experienced include gastrointestinal, pain, sexual disorders, pseudoneurological symptoms, during the course of illness.

    ———

667. Which of the following statements about denial is **false?**

    a. Denial may be either adaptive or maladaptive.
    b. Denial often stems from fear of illness and its consequences.
    c. Denial typically represents an abnormal response to an acute stress, such as life-threatening illness.
    d. Even highly functional adults use denial to cope with anxiety or fear.
    e. Patients may deny in order to protect their physicians from feelings of impotence or grief.

    ———

Questions 668-672 are **true-false** *questions.*

668. A patient may be non-compliant with a physician's recommendations without being in denial.

    ———

669. Anosognosia, or unawareness of a neurological deficit, stems from left-sided parietal lesions.

    ———

670. Elderly persons and their families tend to over-report their symptoms and to blame them on advancing age.

    ———

671. Obstacles to interviewing the geriatric patient include cognitive decline, vague complaints, and sensory impairments.

    ———

672. Measures of activities of daily living (ADLs) are useful in the assessment of functional independence of patients.

    ———

673. Which of the following is **not** generally considered to be a basic activity of daily living?

    a. Bathing
    b. Dressing
    c. Feeding
    d. Shopping
    e. Toileting

    ———

674. **True-False.** The Mini Mental State Examination (MMSE) accurately assesses function of the parietal and frontal lobes.

    ———

675. Which of the following statements about psychological responses to cancer is *false?*

a. A variably depressed mood in the first month after the diagnosis is abnormal.
b. Complete denial of the diagnosis prevents the patient from considering responsible or reasonable choices.
c. Hypervigilance and an all-consuming preoccupation with the resulting diagnosis constitutes an abnormal response.
d. Patients may initially deny or not believe the diagnosis of cancer.
e. Worrying enough to seek medical advice about a physical symptom and the possibility of having cancer is adaptive.

_____

676. Which of the following is a hormonal therapy for cancer?
a. 5-fluouricil
b. Interferon
c. Paclitaxel
d. Procarbazine
e. Tamoxifen

_____

677. Which of the following is *least* likely as a side effect of corticosteroids?

a. Complex partial seizures
b. Depression
c. Emotional lability
d. Insomnia
e. Mania

_____

678. Which of the following is *least* likely to cause akathisia?

a. Aminoglutethimide
b. Droperidol
c. Metoclopramide
d. Perphenazine
e. Prochlorperazine

_____

679. Which of the following statements about hypercalcemia is *false?*

a. Hypercalcemia causes anorexia.
b. Hypercalcemia causes impaired concentration.
c. Hypercalcemia causes lethargy.
d. Hypercalcemia causes tetany.
e. Hypercalcemia is associated with metastatic disease.

_____

680. Which of the following is *not* a common cause of delirium in patients with cancer?

a. Electrolyte imbalance
b. Hypoxia
c. Metastatic lesions in the brain
d. Psychological reactions to the diagnosis of cancer
e. Use of opiates and anticholinergic medications

_____

681. Which of the following statements about paraneoplastic syndromes is *false?*

    a. Paraneoplastic syndromes are associated with delirious states.
    b. Paraneoplastic syndromes are associated with increased ADH secretion and hyponatremia.
    c. Paraneoplastic syndromes are associated with lesions in the cerebral cortex.
    d. Paraneoplastic syndromes are associated with increased parathyroid hormone.
    e. Paraneoplastic syndromes are associated with increased ACTH and Cushing's syndrome.

    _____

682. Which of the following is *not* considered a treatment for post-chemotherapy nausea and vomiting?

    a. Dexamethasone
    b. Droperidol
    c. Ondansetron
    d. Prochlorperazine
    e. Sumatriptan

    _____

683. Which of the following is thought to be ondansetron's mechanism of action?

    a. Cholinergic agonism
    b. Dopaminergic agonism
    c. Dopaminergic antagonism
    d. Serotonergic agonism
    e. Serotonergic antagonism

    _____

684. Which of the following is thought to be metaclopramide's mechanism of action?

    a. Cholinergic agonism
    b. Dopaminergic agonism
    c. Dopaminergic antagonism
    d. Serotonergic agonism
    e. Serotonergic antagonism

    _____

685. Which of the following is *not* a function of palliative care?

    a. Attendance to spiritual concerns
    b. Facilitating the end of life with the use of narcotics
    c. Maintenance of day-to-day activities necessary for sustaining a comforting home environment
    d. Maintenance or repair of family and other interpersonal relationships
    e. Provision of symptom control

    _____

*Questions 686-690 are **true-false** questions.*

686. When receiving palliative care, continued aggressive treatment is not clinically or ethically appropriate for the terminally ill.

    _____

687. The amount of information provided to an adult patient with a terminal illness is determined by the patient's spouse.

    _____

688. The neuropsychiatric complications of terminal illness are commonly recognized and treated.

_____

689. Depression has been estimated to occur in up to 15% of patients with a terminal illness.

_____

690. Nearly 30% of patients develop delirium near the end of life.

_____

691. Which of the following statements about the use of psychostimulants in patients with terminal illness is *false?*

    a. Dextroamphetamine should be avoided because of its high potential for abuse.
    b. Methylphenidate is often prescribed in doses of 2.5 to 20 mg b.i.d. to treat depressive symptoms.
    c. Psychostimulants have a rapid onset of action.
    d. Psychostimulants may precipitate agitation or delirium in susceptible patients.
    e. Tolerance to psychostimulants may develop requiring a dose increase.

_____

692. Which of the following statements related to the breaking of bad news is *false?*

    a. Compassionate communication can make an enormous difference for patients and their families.
    b. It is best for the physician to sit down with the patient or family member when about to deliver bad news.
    c. It is best to give detailed descriptions of the situation when delivering bad news.
    d. It is important to concentrate on listening as much as speaking.
    e. The physician must bear the consequences of being a messenger of ill tidings.

_____

*Questions 693-694 are **true-false** questions.*

693. Mourning for our offspring is generally more difficult than mourning for our elders or our parents.

_____

694. Physicians should urge parents to get over a perinatal death as quickly as possible and to help the parents get on with attempts to conceive again.

_____

695. When learning about bad news or of serious or life-threatening illness, which of the following is *not* a common concern of the patient?

    a. An impending loss of dignity associated with terminal illness
    b. Concern about how to tell others about their illness
    c. Survival until they can witness an important milestone
    d. The physician's belief that the illness was the result of an unhealthy lifestyle
    e. The loss of earning capacity and anticipated medical expenses

    ———

696. Which of the following is generally *not* experienced by physicians who deliver bad news about life-threatening illness to patients?

    a. A feeling of catastrophic loss
    b. A sense of guilt and excessive responsibility
    c. A sense of helplessness
    d. A sense of failure
    e. Feelings of grief

    ———

Questions 697-702 are true-false questions.

697. Withholding and withdrawing life-sustaining treatment can be both morally and legally permissible.

    ———

698. In physician-assisted suicide, the physician administers a medication to a patient to end their suffering.

    ———

699. Giving large doses of narcotics to decrease pain or to ease dyspnea, even if it shortens life, is not considered euthanasia.

    ———

700. Only a judge can declare a patient to be incompetent.

    ———

701. Health care proxies can overrule the decisions of a competent patient.

    ———

702. A competent adult patient has the legal right to refuse treatment even if that decision will lead to harm.

    ———

703. Which of the following statements about grief is *false?*

    a. Acute grief is the first phase of the bereavement process.
    b. Grief is an abnormal response to feeling lost and bereaved.
    c. Grief is not limited to loss by a death though it may follow any recent loss, injury, illness, or disenfranchisement.
    d. Grief is usually proportionate to the disruption caused by loss.
    e. Seldom does acute grief pose a medical or a psychiatric emergency.

    ———

704. Which of the following statements about acute grief is *false?*

   a. As a rule, statements made by well-meaning friends and family unwittingly attempt to abort the mourning process.
   b. Death of a person or a relationship disapproved of by society may still lead to grief.
   c. Frequently intervention depends on a balance between acceptance of a loss and denial of it.
   d. Grief, in general, lasts for several weeks.
   e. In general, sayings like "Try to control yourself" are ineffective and counter-productive.

705. Which of the following statements about pain is *false?*

   a. All pain has a psychological component.
   b. Pain is an unpleasant sensory and emotional experience arising from actual or potential tissue damage.
   c. Pain is one of the most common symptoms reported to physicians.
   d. Patients in pain often fear becoming addicted to analgesics.
   e. Pain is usually diagnosed by use of objective tests.

Questions 706 through 709 involve matching the terms in the left-hand column with the definitions in the right-hand column.

706. _____ Allodynia

707. _____ Hyperpathia

708. _____ Hyperesthesia

709. _____ Hyperalgesia

   a. An increased response to a stimulus that is normally painful

   b. An exaggerated pain response to a noxious stimulus

   c. Pain from a sensation not normally painful

   d. Pain from painful stimuli with delay and persistence beyond stimulation

710. Which of the following statements about reflex sympathetic dystrophy (RSD) is *false?*

a. Pain, edema, and warm skin may last up to 6 months in RSD.

b. RSD is a syndrome of pain in an extremity mediated by sympathetic overactivity that does not involve a major nerve.

c. RSD is a syndrome with sensory, autonomic, and motor features.

d. RSD is usually caused by a major injury.

e. Spontaneous pain occurs in a majority of cases of RSD.

_____

711. Which of the following is *not* equipotent in analgesic effect to 10 mg of parenteral morphine sulfate?

a. Oral codeine 130 mg

b. Oral hydromorphone 7.5 mg

c. Parenteral hydromorphone 1.5 mg

d. Parenteral meperidine 100 mg

e. Parenteral methadone 20 mg

_____

712. According to DSM-IV criteria, dementia involves an acquired deficit in memory and at least one other area of higher cortical function. Which of the following is *not* one of the areas on that list?

a. Agnosia

b. Aphasia

c. Aprosodia

d. Apraxia

e. Executive dysfunction (e.g., impairment of abstraction or planning)

_____

Questions 713 through 717 require matching of the columns.

713. _____Agnosia is

714. _____Apraxia is

715. _____Aphasia is

716. _____Acalculia is

717. _____Aprosodia is

a. An inability to carry out motor tasks despite intact motor function

b. A failure to recognize familiar objects despite intact sensory function

c. A difficulty with language

d. An inability to interpret emotional cues or to convey them

e. An inability to calculate

718. Which of the following statements about dementia is *false?*

   a. By age 85, the prevalence may be as high as 25%.
   b. Dementia is associated with significant impairment in social or occupational function.
   c. Homozygote apolipoprotein E4 alleles occur more commonly in patients with dementia of the Alzheimer's type than those without it.
   d. Not all dementias are progressive.
   e. The prevalence of dementia in those over the age of 60 is 15%.

   _____

*Questions 719 and 720 are **true-false** questions.*

719. Pick's disease primarily affects the temporal lobes.

   _____

720. Creutzfeldt-Jakob disease is a slowly progressive disorder caused by a prion.

   _____

Questions 721 through 725 involve matching the brain region on the left-hand column with the behavior listed in the right-hand column.

721. _____ Frontal   a. Abulia

722. _____ Parietal   b. Extrapyramidal movement disorder

723. _____ Temporal   c. Sensory aprosodia

724. _____ Thalamus   d. Confabulation

725. _____ Striatum   e. Finger agnosia

Questions 726 through 730 involve matching the type of aphasia in the left-hand column with the manifestations of it in the right-hand column.

726. _____ Global

727. _____ Wernicke's

728. _____ Broca's

729. _____ Conduction

730. _____ Transcortical motor

a. Repetition impaired, comprehension intact, speech nonfluent

b. Repetition impaired, comprehension intact, speech fluent

c. Repetition impaired, comprehension impaired, speech nonfluent

d. Repetition intact, comprehension intact, speech nonfluent

e. Repetition impaired, comprehension impaired, speech fluent

Questions 731 through 735 involve matching the terms used in the left-hand column with the definition listed in the right-hand column.

731. _____ Dysnomia

732. _____ Alexia

733. _____ Abulia

734. _____ Dyspraxia

735. _____ Echopraxia

a. Involuntary imitation of movements made by another person

b. Difficulty executing purposeful movements, such as brushing the teeth

c. Lack of motivation to speak, move, or act

d. Word-finding difficulty

e. Inability to comprehend written material

736. Which type of hallucination is typically associated with the Charles Bonnet syndrome?
    a. Auditory
    b. Gustatory
    c. Olfactory
    d. Tactile
    e. Visual

_____

*Questions 737-739 are **true-false** questions.*

737. All complex partial seizures originate in the temporal lobe.

_____

738. An aura is a simple partial seizure with sensory or autonomic phenomena that may develop into a complex partial seizure with or without secondary generalization.

_____

739. The duration of a pseudo-seizure is typically longer than that of a generalized seizure.

_____

740. Which of the following statements about closed-head injuries is *false?*

    a. Acceleration and deceleration forces may cause significant neuronal damage from sheer forces.
    b. A majority of symptoms experienced by patients in the initial phase post-concussion resolve by 3-6 months.
    c. Closed-head injuries result from non-penetrating blows to the head with or without loss of consciousness.
    d. The primary brain injury in closed-head injury typically occurs in the anterior temporal lobes and the inferior surface of the frontal lobes.
    e. The yearly incidence of brain injury following concussive syndromes secondary to closed-head injury is roughly the same as in stroke.

_____

741. Which of the following statements about treatment strategies related to brain-injured patients is *false?*

    a. Behavioral techniques help manage aggressive outbursts and inappropriate social behavior.
    b. Brain-injured patients tolerate neuroleptics as well as non-brain-injured patients.
    c. Family therapy and couple's counseling may be helpful when dealing with personality changes following brain injury.
    d. Following closed-head injury, aggressive behavior may respond to antidepressants, buspirone, anticonvulsants, neuroleptics, and beta-blockers.
    e. Vocational counseling and skills retraining may be helpful to work around deficits.

Questions 742 through 752 are true-false questions.

742. CT is contraindicated in pregnancy.

---

743. In neuroimaging studies, T-1 weighted images are useful to detect areas of pathology.

---

744. CT is superior to MRI for visualization of the posterior fossa and the brainstem.

---

745. The absence of nocturnal penile tumescence (NPT) suggests an organic etiology for impotence.

---

746. Erectile dysfunction is another name for Peyronni's disease.

---

747. The strongest predictor of post-partum depression is affective disturbance during pregnancy.

---

748. When the frequency of congenital malformation after prenatal exposure to a medication is increased compared with the baseline incidence of congenital malformations without such drug exposure, a drug is labeled a teratogen.

---

749. Prenatal exposure to lithium carbonate during the first 12 weeks of gestation is associated with a risk for Goldstein's anomaly.

---

750. Use of valproic acid is associated with less than a 2% to 3% risk of neural tube defects following first trimester exposure.

---

751. Postpartum psychosis is a rare condition that occurs in one to two of every 1,000 post-partum women.

---

752. Breast-feeding while the mother is taking lithium is not recommended.

---

753. At any point in time, what percentage of those diagnosed with bipolar disorder are receiving medical treatment?

    a. Less than 10%
    b. 15%-20%
    c. 25%-30%
    d. 35%-40%
    e. Greater than 50%

    ———

754. Causes of secondary mania include each of the following conditions *except:*

    a. HIV infection
    b. Hypercalcemia
    c. Multiple sclerosis
    d. Systemic lupus erythematosus
    e. Thyrotoxicosis

    ———

755. Prior to lithium therapy, laboratory tests often recommended include each of the following *except:*

    a. BUN and creatinine
    b. Complete blood count
    c. Electrolytes
    d. Liver function tests
    e. Thyroid function tests

    ———

756. Which of the following features or conditions is *least* likely to be associated with bulimia nervosa?

    a. Abrasions on the metacarpopharyngeal joints (Russell's sign)
    b. Lanugo (fine hair on the face and arms)
    c. Parotidomegaly
    d. Perimolysis (enamel loss)
    e. Signs of dehydration

    ———

*Questions 757-759 are **true-false** questions.*

757. HIV infects the brain early in the course of infection, but the frequency and severity of clinically important HIV CNS infections generally parallels those of systemic HIV disease.

    ———

758. Use of psychostimulants (e.g., dextroamphetamine and methylphenidate) may reduce the symptoms of decreased attention and concentration as well as apathetic mood in those with HIV infection.

    ———

759. Painful peripheral neuropathies commonly result from HIV infection and the neurotoxic side effects of nucleoside anti-retroviral agents.

    ———

760. Which of the following statements about noncompliance is *false* regarding patients undergoing organ transplantation?

    a. Noncompliance is difficult to predict.
    b. Noncompliance may present as missed medication, missed appointments, or a patient's failure to make a timely report of important symptomatic changes.
    c. Noncompliance is not a reason to exclude a patient from a transplant list.
    d. Great distances from a transplant center may increase the chance for noncompliance.
    e. Assessment of noncompliance involves knowledge of cognitive deficits, presence of depression, and prior noncompliance.

    _____

*Questions 761 and 762 are **true-false** questions.*

761. In general, difficulty in treating celebrities occurs not because they are entitled, demanding, or seductive but because of the publicity that surrounds them.

    _____

762. Multiple visits to an emergency room for any reason should raise one's concern that the patient is being abused.

    _____

763. Signs and symptoms of opiate withdrawal typically include each of the following *except:*

    a. Decreased respiratory rate
    b. Dilated pupils
    c. Lacrimation
    d. Rhinorrhea
    e. Yawning

    _____

764. Life-threatening causes of agitation include each of the following *except:*

    a. Hypoglycemia
    b. Hypertension
    c. Intracranial bleeding
    d. Meningitis
    e. Normal pressure hydrocephalus

    _____

765. Life-threatening causes of agitation include each of the following *except:*

    a. General paresis
    b. Hypoxia
    c. Poisoning
    d. Wernicke's encephalopathy
    e. Withdrawal from barbiturates

    _____

766. When interviewing and examining a violent or potentially violent patient, useful strategies include each of the following *except:*

    a. Accept what the patient tells you
    b. Agree to whatever they ask for to avoid a crisis
    c. Attend to the patient's physical comfort
    d. Express concern for the patient
    e. Use a calm, nonthreatening language

    _____

767. **True-False**. When interviewing the potentially violent patient, it is best to be nonthreatening and to interview the patient alone so as not to threaten the patient by the presence of security personnel.

_____

768. Which of the following statements about glucocorticoid treatments is *false?*

a. Among the patients who develop psychiatric complications secondary to glucocorticoid treatment, roughly 40% develop symptoms in the first week of treatment.
b. Most patients recover from their psychiatric symptoms within 6 weeks of discontinuation of glucocorticoids.
c. Neuropsychiatric symptoms generally start after several months of ongoing glucocorticoid treatment.
d. Roughly 5% of glucocorticoid-treated patients develop severe psychiatric syndromes including depression, mania, psychosis, and delirium.
e. Up to 30% of glucocorticoid-treated patients develop at least mild psychiatric symptoms.

_____

769. **True-False**. A history of psychiatric illness is a clear risk factor for the development of psychiatric symptoms from glucocorticoids.

_____

770. Approximately what percent of patients receiving more than 80 mg per day of prednisone will develop neuropsychiatric side-effects?

a. Less than 1%
b. 1%-5%
c. 5%-15%
d. 15%-25%
e. Greater than 50%

_____

771. Which of the following *most* often causes orthostatic hypotension?

a. Bupropion
b. Fluoxetine
c. Mirtazapine
d. Nortriptyline
e. Phenelzine

_____

772. The American Medical Association's Council on Ethical and Judicial Affairs passed a rule that prohibited physician/patient sexual contact regardless of the physician's specialty.

_____

773. Inappropriate behavior during a physical examination can lead to civil and potentially criminal litigation.

_____

774. Which of the following *most* often causes prolongation of the QRS interval?

a. Bupropion
b. Fluoxetine
c. Imipramine
d. Phenelzine
e. Trazodone

_____

775. Which of the following is the *least* sedating?

    a. Bupropion
    b. Clomipramine
    c. Doxepin
    d. Mirtazapine
    e. Trazodone

    ―――――――

776. MAOI-induced paresthesias may be treated by which of the following?

    a. Amantadine
    b. Cyproheptadine
    c. Pyridoxine
    d. Trazodone
    e. Zolpidem

    ―――――――

Questions 777-791 are true-false questions.

777. All TCAs prolong the His-Ventricular (H-V) interval and increase the risk of orthostatic hypotension in the presence of bundle branch block.

    ―――――――

778. Lithium levels remain stable when thiazide diuretics are administered.

    ―――――――

779. Torsades de pointes is another name for hyperacute T waves.

    ―――――――

780. Medications with a narrow therapeutic window are relatively ineffective above a specified therapeutic range.

    ―――――――

781. Idiosyncratic reactions are rare but predictable reactions given knowledge of pharmacokinetics and pharmacodynamic properties.

    ―――――――

782. Common inhibitors of hepatic metabolic enzymes include ketoconazole, cimetidine, erythromycin, and phenytoin.

    ―――――――

783. Inhibitors of hepatic metabolic enzymes typically produce an abrupt elevation in the blood levels of the co-administered drug.

    ―――――――

784. Discontinuation of an inhibitor of hepatic metabolic enzymes is associated with a rapid fall in blood levels of a co-administered drug.

    ―――――――

785. Inducers of hepatic metabolic enzymes produce an abrupt decline in the blood levels of the co-administered drug.

    ―――――――

786. Addition of an ACE inhibitor to lithium decreases lithium levels.

    ―――――――

787. Informed consent is a process through which the physician gets the permission of a patient or a substituted decision-maker to provide treatment to that patient.

    ―――――――

788. A physician who obtains informed consent in a reasonable way is less likely to be perceived as arrogant and deserving of a law suit by distressed patients if an adverse outcome develops.

_____

789. When a competent patient wishes to pass the right to make a decision to a family member or to the physician, the patient may do so.

_____

790. Only a psychiatrist can declare a patient to be incompetent.

_____

791. The conclusion that a patient lacks the capacity to give informed consent requires the choice of an alternative decision maker except in an emergency or when the patient has a valid advanced directive.

_____

792. When a physician evaluates a patient's capacity to make treatment decisions, each of the following questions is crucial *except:*

a. Can the patient manipulate the information provided in a rational fashion as to how a decision that follows is logical from the information in the control of the individual's personal beliefs, experience, and condition?
b. Does the patient express a preference?
c. Does the patient have minor children?
d. Is the patient able to attain a factual understanding of the information provided?
e. Is the patient able to appreciate the seriousness of the condition and the consequences of accepting or refusing treatment?

_____

*Questions 793-800 are **true-false** questions.*

793. Patients who are unable to express a preference are presumed to lack decision-making capacity.

_____

794. Disagreement with the treating clinician and his or her recommendations is and of itself not a basis for judging that a patient is irrational.

_____

795. In an emergency, informed consent need not be obtained.

_____

796. If a patient's physical or mental condition will deteriorate as a direct result of the process of providing information, informed consent may be deferred under the doctrine of therapeutic privilege.

———

797. The patient or decision-maker may withdraw consent at any point during the course of treatment.

———

798. In most states, involuntary commitment of a patient allows for the treatment of a patient against his/her will.

———

799. All adults, even those with mental illness, are presumed to be competent.

———

800. In many states, the law imposes a duty on clinicians to take steps to protect the safety of third parties against whom a patient issues threats.

———

Answers

1. The answer is **a**. Many believe that James Eaton was responsible for the growth of C-L Psychiatry by his funding of C-L programs. James Putnam was a young Harvard neurologist who was appointed as "electrician" at the Massachusetts General Hospital (MGH) in 1873. Howard Means was Chief of Medicine at the MGH in the 1920s; he appointed William Herman to study patients with mental disturbances in conjunction with endocrine disorders. Thomas Hackett was Chief of the MGH Psychiatric Consultation Service and then Chief of the Department of Psychiatry at the MGH until the time of his death in 1988. Though influential through is role at the MGH and his work with the Academy of Psychosomatic Medicine, Hackett did not work at the NIMH.

2. The answer is **c**. Bibring and Deutsch were among a number of European immigrants with psychoanalytic training who fled Nazi Germany for the safety of the United States. Avery Weisman, who was the first Chief of the Psychiatric Consultation Service at the MGH, and Thomas Hackett, Weisman's first resident, created, in 1956, a service that thrives today. But it was Erich Lindemann who performed the classic study on victims of the Coconut Grove Fire.

3. The answer is **d**.

4. The answer is **a**.

5. The answer is **e**.

6. The answer is **c**.

7. The answer is **b**. Broca, who lived from 1824 to 1880, is best known for his work on aphasia, in part derived from his work with Monsieur Laborgne. His brain rests in the L'Ecole de Medicine in Paris, next to Laborgne's brain.

8. The answer is **false**. It was Sperry, not Brodmann. Sperry's work led to the conclusion that many things can happen affectually without all of the neocortex being cognizant of what is occurring.

9. The answer is **true**. Analogous to the tail of a dog whose tail-wagging frequency and vigor can tell us about the dog's feelings, the smile services that function in humans.

10. The answer is **e**. Another way of conceptualizing the function of the limbic system is to view it, as Murray says, mediating the four Fs: fear, feeding, fighting, and fornicating. The limbic system lacks words, but it is instrumental in allowing the individual to feel one's affect.

11. The answer is **e**. Brodmann's area # 17 is part of the primary visual cortex in the occipital lobe. The other areas mentioned are part of Papez's circuit of the limbic system.

12. The answer is **d**. In fact, they tend to be vigilant about avoiding

emotional extremes that could impair judgment.

13. The answer is **c**. Bad copers often find it difficult to weigh feasible alternatives and fail to initiate action on their own behalf.

14. The answer is **true**. Vulnerability is present in all humans and appears at times of crisis.

15. The answer is **b**. Depression accounts for approximately 23% of total psychiatric admissions. An estimated 80% of persons with depression are either treated by non-psychiatric personnel or go untreated.

16. The answer is **false**. Major depression is not an appropriate reaction to illness. Major depression is not solely a reaction with sadness or despondency, but a serious condition capable of endangering the patient. Depression is a dread complication of medical illness that requires diagnosis and treatment.

17. The answer is **true**. The DSM-IV criteria for major depression, with presence of five or more of the nine neurovegetative symptoms of depression being present most of the day for nearly every day, including depressed mood or a loss of interest, are the same for the medically ill as for the non-medically ill.

18. The answer is **true**. Patients with coronary artery disease and depression are more likely to have ventricular tachycardia and a higher rate of reduced heart rate variability, each of which increases the risk of sudden death.

19. The answer is **false**. Left untreated, major depression lasts about one year, but minor depression lasts approximately two years.

20. The answer is **false**. Aprosodia (the lack of prosody or inflection, rhythm, and intensity of expression) which occurs when the right hemisphere is damaged, may be a sequela of stroke but it does not in and of itself cause major depression.

21. The answer is **false**. It does, but not as much as does multi-infarct dementia or vascular dementia.

22. The answer is **true**. However, trazodone, which has low affinity for this H_1 receptor, is sedating.

23. The answer is **true**. Weight gain is correlated with histamine H_1 receptor affinity.

24. The answer is **false**. Just the reverse is true. Doxepin is an exceedingly potent antihistamine.

25. The answer is **true**. Amitriptyline does have a greater affinity for muscarinic receptors than does protriptyline.

26. The answer is **false**. Orthostatic hypotension is not directly related to α_1 noradrenergic receptor affinity.

27. The answer is **true**.

28. The answer is **true**.

29. The answer is **false**. Sinus tachycardia may result from muscarinic blockade of vagal tone in the heart.

30. The answer is **false**. Cardiac transplantation denervates the heart, which prevents the usual muscarinic blockade-enhancing effects of vagal tone by TCAs.

31. The answer is **false**. Suppression of appetite by psychostimulants is exceedingly uncommon among the depressed medically ill. In fact, psychostimulants usually enhance the appetite of these patients.

32. The answer is **false**. T-wave flattening, a benign and reversible phenomenon, is seen in approximately 50% of cases.

33. The answer is **true**. For every person who completes suicide, 8-10 people attempt suicide.

34. The answer is **false**. Use of firearms is the most common method of committing suicide.

35. The answer is **true**. Drug overdose is the second most common method used by women and hanging is the second most common method used by men who attempt suicide.

36. The answer is **true**. Those greater than 65 years of age are one and a half times more likely to commit suicide than are younger individuals.

37. The answer is **false**. One of every four attempts in this group results in suicide.

38. The answer is **false**. Women are four times more likely to commit suicide than are men.

39. The answer is **true**. Native Americans and Alaskan natives have the highest rate of suicide, while African American and Hispanics have approximately one-half the suicide rate of whites in the United States.

40. The answer is **true**. Alcohol and drug abuse are associated with sui-cide, with more serious attempts, and with a greater number of attempts.

41. The answer is **false**. The suicide risk is 16-66 times greater in AIDS patients than it is in those in the general population.

42. The answer is **false**. Head trauma is associated with a suicide risk that is two times that of the general population. The risk increases in those who suffer severe injuries and in those who develop dementia, psychosis, or epilepsy.

43. The answer is **c**. Among these conditions listed, patients with chronic renal failure who receive hemodialysis have a rate of suicide that may be as high as 400 times that of the general population.

44. The answer is **false**. The evaluation of suicide is an emergent procedure, and risk of suicide takes precedence over the desire of the patient for privacy and the maintenance of confidentiality in the physician/patient relationship.

45. The answer is **true**. Patients at potential risk of suicide, and who threaten to leave before an adequate evaluation is complete, must be detained in accordance with the state statutes that permit detention and evaluation of patients in danger of harming themselves or others.

46. Answer is **true**. Patients who are at high risk of suicide, and who refuse hospitalization, should be committed involuntarily.

47. The answer is **c**. Symptoms of depression are predictors of response to electroconvulsive therapy (ECT). Sustained improvement of

drug-resistant chronic schizophrenia may be achieved with ECT. Greater than 50% of drug-refractory mania is effectively treated with ECT, and the majority of such patients respond promptly. However, posttraumatic stress disorder is not among the conditions listed as being ECT-responsive.

48. The answer is **false**. Transient bradycardia and hypotension often occur during the time period 5-10 minutes following ECT, while parasympathetic activity remains strong.

49. The answer is **e**. Appropriate monitoring of blood pressure is required during, and following, ECT.

50. The answer is **true**. In fact, Parkinson's disease, even in the absence of depression, may be an indication for ECT.

51. The answer is **false**. Depressed pregnant women with severe depression may require ECT to prevent malnutrition or suicide. The fetus may be protected from physiological stress during ECT by virtue of its lack of direct neuronal connection to the maternal diencephalon.

52. The answer is **false**. Benzodiazepines are antagonistic to the ictal process and should be discontinued prior to ECT. Even short-acting benzodiazepines may make treatment impossible.

53. The answer is **d**. CXR, ECG, CBC, and serum electrolytes are indicated tests, while an ESR, a general screen for inflammation, is not. Also indicated are determinations of serum glucose, blood urea nitrogen (BUN), and, at the discretion of the clinician, a more complete cognitive assessment of the patient.

54. The answer is **true**. This recommendation was endorsed by the American Society of Anesthesiologists.

55. The answer is **false**. These agents, atropine and glycopyrrolate, are not routinely administered because they increase cardiac work during treatment and do not decrease oral secretions.

56. The answer is **b**. Typically, short-acting intravenous agents (e.g., esmolol or labetalol) are given immediately before the anesthetic induction. They may worsen, not reduce, CHF.

57. The answer is **true**. Unilateral ECT, when ineffective, is associated with use of threshold stimulus intensity and a short distance between the electrodes.

58. The answer is **false**. Brief-pulse wave forms have become the standard of practice in the United States because they more effectively induce seizure activity and are associated with less post-treatment confusion and amnesia.

59. The answer is **true**. Seizure generalization can be monitored by inflation of a blood pressure cuff on the arm or ankle above systolic pressure just before injection of succinylcholine. The convulsion can then be observed in the unparalyzed extremity.

60. The answer is **a**. Advanced age is associated with more problems than is experienced by younger patients, the group to which pregnant women belong.

61. The answer is **c**. The diagnostic criteria are disturbance of consciousness, a change in cognition not better accounted for by a pre-existing or established or evolving dementia, a disturbance that develops over a short period of time and which tends to fluctuate, and evidence that the disturbance is caused by the direct physiological consequence of a general medical condition.

62. The answer is **true**. Impaired attention is more significant than is the level of psychomotor activity.

63. The answer is **false**. The term intensive care unit (ICU) psychosis is often applied to patients with abnormal behavior in the ICU and erroneously attributed to sensory deprivation or overload.

64. The answer is **false**. Adrenergic delirium (e.g., as caused by hypoglycemia) most commonly presents with moist skin and tachycardia, whereas a patient with an anticholinergic delirium presents with dry skin and tachycardia.

65. The answer is **true**. Physostigmine, an anticholinergic esterase, has been successfully used to diagnose and treat anticholinergic delirium.

66. The answer is **c**. Other conditions to assess include intracranial hemorrhage, meningitis or encephalitis, and poisonings.

67. The answer is **true**. Seriously ill hospitalized patients often suffer encephalopathy when bacteremic.

68. The answer is **false**. A host of conditions other than delirium are associated with very low MMSE scores, including coma and dementia.

69. The answer is **d**. Motor function, as opposed to frontal function, is associated with observation of drift.

70. The answer is **false**. Serial 7s tests for attention and calculation ability.

71. The answer is **false**. Not all cases of delirium require neuroleptics. Treatment is dependent upon the nature of the problem (e.g., discontinuation of the offending agent and replacement of a specific antidote).

72. The answer is **d**. Accumulation of the active CNS metabolite of meperidine, normeperidine, commonly causes mental status changes and myoclonus.

73. The answer is **true**. While not approved for use by the intravenous route, haloperidol has been used this way for more than 30 years.

74. The answer is **true**. When either of these agents is co-administered through the IV line, the IV line must first be flushed with saline to prevent precipitation.

75. The answer is **b**.

76. The answer is **e**.

77. The answer is **a**.

78. The answer is **d**.

79. The answer is **c**. Whenever possible, delirium should be treated by removal of the offending agent and by reversal with a specific antidote.

80. The answer is **true**. To prevent seizures, IV dosing should be slowly administered over 1-2 minutes using low doses, such as 0.5 mg to 1 mg to start.

81. The answer is **true**. This anticholinergic agent does not cross the blood brain barrier and should protect the patient from peripheral cholinergic actions of physostigmine.

82. The answer is **true**. In contrast to the immediately observable effects of IV diazepam, IV haloperidol has a distribution time of 11 minutes.

83. The answer is **false**. Just the opposite is true. IV haloperidol causes extrapyramidal effects less often than does IM administration.

84. The answer is **true**. While the mechanism of action is unclear, several case reports have associated use of haloperidol with torsades de pointes, a condition that is probably exacerbated by low levels of potassium and magnesium, by prolongation of the QT interval, as well as by hepatic compromise or specific cardiac abnormalities.

85. The answer is **true**. However, droperidol is more likely to cause more orthostatic hypotension than is haloperidol, which may make its use in the medically ill less likely.

86. The answer is **true**. Extrapyramidal side effects and neuroleptic malignant syndrome may be more common in HIV-infected patients.

87. The answer is **true**. Propofol delivered as a fat emulsion, can lead to a fat overload syndrome associated with CO_2 production, hypertriglyceridemia, ketoacidosis, seizure activity, and respiratory failure.

88. The answer is **false**. Administration of flumazenil to a benzodiazepine-dependent patient can precipitate seizures.

89. The answer is **false**. Determination of changes in heart rate and blood pressure during the interview and the physical exam may reflect levels of alertness. An increase in heart rate or blood pressure usually indicates that the patient is awake and inadequately sedated.

90. The answer is **c**. A family history is not indicative of a diagnosis of delirium.

91. The answer is **d**. Recent memory is worse than is remote memory in DAT.

92. The answer is **d**. Speech latency is increased with depression.

93. The answer is **c**. Nearly 4 million Americans are affected by dementia; this accounts for 15% of those more than 65 years of age.

94. The answer is **true**. Cognitive deficits in Alzheimer's disease cause significant amounts of social and occupational dysfunction.

95. The answer is **false**. The diagnosis of dementia does not take away someone's rights. Cognitive assessments should be conducted if doubts arise as to whether a demented individual has the capacity to provide consent and to be involved in informed medical decision-making.

96. The answer is **false**. CJD's decline is more rapid than the decline in DAT.

97. The answer is **false**. No, these symptoms are typically present in normal pressure hydrocephalus (NPH).

98. The answer is **d**. Focal neurological findings, depression, and a history of

cerebrovascular accidents (CVAs) are often present in vascular dementia.

99. The answer is **false**. Visual hallucinations are more common than are auditory hallucinations in DAT.

100. The answer is **false**. Capgras syndrome is a syndrome in which the affected individual believes that familiar people have been replaced by impostors.

101. The answer is **false**. The situation described would be an agnosia. An apraxia is the inability to carry out motor tasks despite intact motor systems and an understanding of the task.

102. The answer is **c**.

103. The answer is **d**.

104. The answer is **a**.

105. The answer is **b**.

106. The answer is **e**.

107. The answer is **d**. Of the signs mentioned, Kayser Fleisher rings, which are golden brown deposits circling the cornea, are pathognomonic for the disease.

108. The answer is **false**. At least four weeks of these symptoms must be present for the diagnosis of schizophrenia to be made.

109. The answer is **b**. Low-potency neuroleptics, like thioridazine, tend to have a low prevalence of extrapyramidal symptoms, including dystonia.

110. The answer is **true**. Clozapine is a potent anticholinergic neuroleptic.

111. The answer is **b**. Weight gain and urinary incontinence are associated with atypical neuroleptic agents, e.g., with olanzapine and clozapine treatment.

112. The answer is **false**. Actually it is agranulocytosis, not leukocytosis, that is common, occurring in 1% of patients.

113. The answer is **c**. Low-potency neuroleptics less frequently cause extrapyramidal symptoms and Parkinsonian symptoms than do higher-potency agents.

114. The answer is **true**. However, once present, it may be irreversible.

115. The answer is **d**. It is leukocytosis, not leukopenia, that is a sign of NMS.

116. The answer is **false**. There is no increased risk and there is no clear linkage between these syndromes.

117. The answer is **false**. No; the 2D6 isoenzyme system is generally involved.

118. The answer is **e**. Cardiac effects are not prominent with polydipsia.

119. The answer is **b**. Patients in cardiology practices have a prevalence of anxiety of 10% to 14%, while the prevalence of panic is 6% to 10% in primary care settings and 1% to 2% in the general population.

120. The answer is **b**. When this area of the brain is stimulated, an acute fear response can be elicited. Destruction of the LC can lead to abnormal complacency in the face of threat in primates.

121. The answer is **d**. Depressive symptoms are frequently co-morbid with anxiety disorders.

122. The answer is **false**. Greater than 90% of panic-disordered patients present with somatic complaints.

123. The answer is **true**. Mitral valve prolapse, usually asymptomatic, may predispose to arrhythmia; it occurs in roughly 5% to 10% of the population and in 30% to 50% of those with panic disorder.

124. The answer is **false**. Major depressive disorder occurs in approximately two-thirds of all cases of panic disorder.

125. The answer is **true**. Because of their broad spectrum of efficacy, favorable side-effect profile, and lack of cardiotoxicity, SSRIs have become a first-line treatment for panic disorder.

126. The answer is **true**. At times, SSRIs may worsen anxiety at initiation of treatment. Thus, patients should be started at one-half or less of the usual starting dose.

127. The answer is **false**. Treatment response usually develops after 2-3 weeks of its use.

128. The answer is **false**. Most patients benefit from alprazolam doses of 4 to 8 mg qd for panic disorder.

129. The answer is **false**. Alprazolam's half-life is 12 to 15 hours, while for clonazepam it is 15 to 50 hours.

130. The answer is **false**. While midazolam is a benzodiazepine and is anxiolytic, it is not a standard, or even common, treatment for panic disorder; without an available oral preparation, it requires administration parenterally and has a half-life of 1 to 12 hours.

131. The answer is **false**. While buspirone is used to treat anxiety, buspirone is not a benzodiazepine.

132. The answer is **true**. Controlled studies have demonstrated this finding. As a result, the Institute of Medicine called for screening for alcohol problems with every hospitalized patient.

133. The answer is **false**. Alcohol is a GABA agonist.

134. The answer is **true**. Conversely, successful interviews tend to accept the drunk as he/she is; a handshake of introduction often helps initiate contact.

135. The answer is **false**. More than momentary eye contact is often taken as a challenge and may become the prelude to combat.

136. The answer is **false**. In pathologic intoxication, the patient becomes intoxicated on small amounts of alcohol (e.g., as little as 4 ounces). Automatic behavior and violence may occur for which the patient is amnestic, but hallucinations are not typical.

137. The answer is **false**. Usually, alcohol withdrawal, seizures, or rum fits occur within the first 2 days after stoppage of alcohol.

138. The answer is **true**. Alcoholic hallucinosis may occur during active drinking. However, it typically develops 1-2 days after alcohol cessation.

139. The answer is **false**. Alcohol withdrawal seizures occur in approximately 1% of unmedicated withdrawing alcoholics.

140. The answer is **false**. It is Korsakoff's psychosis that is manifest by confabulation and memory problems.

141. The answer is **true**. Roughly 20% of cases improve more or less completely despite its reputation as conveying a gloomy prognosis.

142. The answer is **b**. Dysarthria is not a part of Wernicke's encephalopathy.

143. The answer is **false**. Thiamine should be administered to prevent an irreversible and incapacitating amnestic disorder. Folic acid should be administered as well.

144. The answer is **c**. Disulfiram reduces subsequent drinking days in chronic alcoholics in approximately 50% of cases; disulfiram interactions do not include bradycardia.

145. The answer is **c**. The signs and symptoms of acute cocaine intoxication parallel those of amphetamine intoxication.

146. The answer is **b**. Mydriasis (i.e., dilated pupils) is more frequently seen than are small pupils.

147. The answer is **d**. It is low mood and anhedonia, not euphoria, which is usually found with chronic cocaine use.

148. The answer is **c**. It is dilated pupils that are seen in narcotic withdrawal. In addition, tremor, increased respiratory rate, tachycardia, hypertension, nausea, and vomiting occur with opiate withdrawal.

149. The answer is **d**. It is insomnia and hyposomnia that accompanies severe opiate withdrawal.

150. The answer is **b**. Currently, ongoing clinical tests of buprenorphine are evaluating its role as an opiate substitute.

151. The answer is **e**. Clonidine is an α_2 adrenergic agonist that can be started at a dose of 5 mcg/kg/d.

152. The answer is **b**. Depression is more typically seen than is nausea, vomiting, anorexia, or euphoria.

153. The answer is **true**. Seizures may result from administration of flumazenil in those taking TCAs or in those chronically taking benzodiazepines.

154. The answer is **a**. However, if barbiturates are combined with narcotics, pupils may be small or, if secondary anoxia is present, fixed and dilated pupils may result.

155. The answer is **c**. Cross-tolerance exists for agents that are active at the benzodiazepine, barbiturate and alcohol receptor.

156. The answer is **c**. It is alkalinization of the urine, not acidification of the urine that is indicated in barbiturate overdose.

157. The answer is **true**. When assessing a patient's level of dependence to barbiturates by means of the pentobarbital tolerance test, a 200 mg dose of pentobarbital is administered followed by 100 mg doses every hour, watching for signs of mild toxicity to appear.

158. The answer is **c**. Each of the other tests is a clinician-rated instrument.

159. The answer is **false**. The GAF is recorded on Axis V.

160. The answer is **true**. The GAF can also be used for documentation of treatment course over time.

161. The answer is **false**. Even when a patient's condition is influenced by psychosocial factors, psychotropics may be indicated and be useful.

162. The answer is **true**. Each of the above factors is important for education of the patient and to facilitate compliance.

163. The answer is **false**. Cost and tolerability of psychotropics are important factors to discuss with a patient.

164. The answer is **false**. In approximately two-thirds of patients, initial treatment leads to significant improvement.

165. The answer is **true**. When treatment fails, the clinician must determine the adequacy of dosing.

166. The answer is **false**. These features are related to pharmacokinetic processes.

167. The answer is **true**. Enhanced gastric emptying (e.g., with metoclopramide) and diminishing gastrointestinal motility (e.g., with TCAs) facilitate greater contact with, and absorption from, mucosal surfaces into the systemic circulation.

168. The answer is **true**. Such a mechanism might lead to lower plasma levels.

169. The answer is **false**. Lithium is a water-soluble drug.

170. The answer is **e**. Venlafaxine, lithium, and gabapentin each have minimal protein binding.

171. The answer is **b**. Other inducers include carbamazepine, primidone, and alcohol.

172. The answer is **c**. Other inhibitors include paroxetine, sertraline, nefazodone, methylphenidate, diltiazem, verapamil, and alcohol.

173. The answer is **c**. Theophylline promotes diuresis and excretion of lithium, thereby lowering serum lithium levels.

174. The answer is **false**. Acidification of the urine increases the rate of excretion of weak bases.

175. The answer is **true**. This technique can be used in the management of patients with severe phencyclidine (PCP) or amphetamine intoxication.

176. The answer is **true**. Thereby, this technique can be used in cases of barbiturate overdose.

177. The answer is **false**. Gabapentin is primarily excreted by the kidney in an unchanged form.

178. The answer is **b**. Other than molindone, most neuroleptics are highly protein-bound; that is, between 90% to 98% is bound.

179. The answer is **true**. Addition of antihypertensives to risperidone is likely to achieve significant hypotension, especially early on in treatment.

180. The answer is **true**. Use of antacids will interfere with absorption of neuroleptics and lower serum levels.

181. The answer is **true**. Because smoking is an inducer of hepatic isoenzymes, antipsychotic levels will drop when one smokes cigarettes.

182. The answer is **false**. Co-administration of SSRIs and neuroleptics will increase the SSRI level and the

antipsychotic level by virtue of its role as a hepatic-enzyme inhibitor.

183. The answer is **a**. Aminophylline and theophylline will result in lower lithium levels.

184. The answer is **true**. The same interaction occurs with other neuromuscular blockers (e.g., pancuronium) and lithium.

185. The answer is **e**. Lithium is not highly bound to plasma proteins.

186. The answer is **c**. The elimination half-life of valproic acid is approximately 8 hours.

187. The answer is **a**. In contrast to other major anticonvulsants, it does not inhibit hepatic microsomes.

188. The answer is **true**. Dose reduction of valproic acid may be necessary in the patient starting cimetidine.

189. The answer is **true**. Correspondingly, when fluoxetine is discontinued, the risk of sub-therapeutic valproic acid levels exists.

190. The answer is **c**. Several drugs inhibit the metabolism of carbamazepine, including erythromycin, isoniazid, fluoxetine, valproic acid, and calcium channel blockers. Verapamil and diltiazem raise the level of carbamazepine.

191. The answer is **e**. TCAs are well absorbed from the GI tract and are highly protein-bound (85% to 95%).

192. The answer is **d**. Protriptyline, like desipramine and nortriptyline, is a secondary amine and not a tertiary amine.

193. The answer is **true**. Carbamazepine induces hepatic isoenzymes and lowers levels of TCAs.

194. The answer is **true**.

195. The answer is **true**.

196. The answer is **true**. By virtue of cimetidine's inhibitory effects on hepatic isoenzymes, it can raise TCA levels.

197. The answer is **true**. Most of the SSRIs are highly protein-bound; however, venlafaxine is only 20% to 30% protein-bound.

198. The answer is **false**. It is fluvoxamine that is a potent inhibitor of the 1A2 isoenzyme system.

199. The answer is **false**. Just the reverse is true. The gut primarily has MAO-A, while the brain has MAO-B.

200. The answer is **true**.

201. The answer is **true**. By contrast, tranylcypromine's MAO inhibition may not be entirely irreversible.

202. The answer is **true**.

203. The answer is **b**. Nifedipine treats, not causes, hypertensive crises.

204. The answer is **a**. An indirect-acting vasopressor agent, methylphenidate, causes hypertensive crisis, whereas direct sympathomimetic agents are comparatively safe when taken with MAOIs. The α_1-adrenergic antagonist phentolamine treats hypertensive crises.

205. The answer is **b**. Aged cheeses, yeast extracts, over-ripened fruit, aged meats, many red and some

white wines can precipitate hypertensive crisis.

206. The answer is **d**. Meperidine and dextromethorphan can precipitate fatal reactions when co-administered with MAOIs, whereas other narcotics appear to be safer in conjunction with MAOIs.

207. The answer is **d**. Metoclopramide, a dopamine-blocker, might worsen, rather than reduce, drug-induced extrapyramidal side effects.

208. The answer is **b**. Clonidine induces, not relieves, hypotension. Other helpful agents have included methylphenidate and T-4.

209. The answer is **d**. In addition, neostigmine, amantadine, and trazodone have been used to control sexual dysfunction induced by SSRIs.

210. The answer is **d**. Just the opposite is true. It may treat akathisia as well.

211. The answer is **c**.

212. The answer is **d**.

213. The answer is **b**.

214. The answer is **e**.

215. The answer is **a**.

216. The answer is **b**. Enjoyment in fooling physicians or taking on the patient role by fabrication of symptoms suggests factitious disorder, not malingering.

217. The answer is **a**. Psychiatric referrals are typically few in number in cases of factitious disorder.

218. The answer is **false**. Psychiatric symptoms (e.g., false complaints of hallucinations or suicidal ideation) can also occur.

219. The answer is **c**. After Asher's 1951 article, nearly 100 Letters to the Editor followed with recommendations for alternative names for the syndrome and tips on how to avoid being fooled by these patients.

220. The answer is **false**. By definition the syndrome is neither intentionally produced nor feigned.

221. The answer is **true**. One of the most common variants of monosymptomatic hypochondriacal psychosis is body dysmorphic disorder.

222. The answer is **true**.

223. The answer is **true**. To make the diagnosis, pain must be bilateral, above and below the waist, and involve the axial cervical spine, chest, or lower back. Criteria require 11/18 (9 bilateral) trigger points, according to the American College of Rheumatology.

224. The answer is **true**.

225. The answer is **c**.

226. The answer is **b**.

227. The answer is **a**.

228. The answer is **true**.

229. The answer is **false**. These patients stir up sadistic wishes in caregivers and these wishes inhibit the setting of effective limits.

230. The answer is **c**. Other primitive defenses used by patients with borderline personality organization are psychotic denial and devaluation.

231. The answer is **false**. This is a definition of splitting. Projective identification consists of taking unwanted aspects of the self, such as cruelty or envy, and wholly ascribing it to another.

232. The answer is **true**.

233. The answer is **d**. Narcissism of the consultant has no place in the management of these patients.

234. The answer is **true**.

235. The answer is **true**.

236. The answer is **false**. The International Association of the Study of Pain defines pain as an unpleasant sensory and emotional experience associated with actual, or potential, tissue damage; or described in terms of such damage.

237. The answer is **a**.

238. The answer is **d**.

239. The answer is **e**.

240. The answer is **b**.

241. The answer is **c**.

242. The answer is **false**. Major depressive disorder is diagnosed in approximately 25% of patients with chronic pain.

243. The answer is **b**. Approximately one-half of patients with chronic pain have a conversion V by responses on the MMPI. It has elements with elevated levels of hypochondriasis and hysteria and a relative absence of depression that accompanies conversion.

244. The answer is **true**.

245. The answer is **false**. A placebo trial only shows whether a patient will be responsive to a placebo. It does not prove that a patient is a malingerer or that response would not occur with an active medication.

246. The answer is **d**. Studies have shown that 38% of individuals are placebo responders.

247. The answer is **true**.

248. The answer is **false**. Step 1 involves NSAIDs, aspirin, or acetaminophen. Step 2 adds codeine to NSAIDs with other adjuvants.

249. The answer is **d**. NSAIDs can raise blood pressure in patients treated with β-blockers and diuretics.

250. The answer is **true**.

251. The answer is **false**; 100 mg of IM meperidine is equivalent to 300 mg of oral meperidine.

252. The answer is **false**. The active metabolite of meperidine is normeperidine and it has a long duration of action, nearly 14 hours.

253. The answer is **d**. Normeperidine toxicity may be exacerbated by renal impairment, but it is not a cause of renal impairment.

254. The answer is **true**. It is even more likely to occur in patients with malignancy or with renal impairment.

255. The answer is **false**. Methadone's analgesic efficacy is 6 hours, far less than its pharmacological half-life of 36 hours.

256. The answer is **false**. Pentazocine and butorphanol are mixed agonist-antagonists.

257. The answer is **false**. The risk of narcotics addiction in medically ill patients is approximately 0.3%.

258. The answer is **false**. The dorsolateral funiculus, not the anterolateral columns, house the serotonergic pathways for pain.

259. The answer is **true**.

260. The answer is **false**. It is lamotrigine that is the only direct glutamate/aspartate antagonist.

261. The answer is **false**. Valproate has been shown to decrease postherpetic neuralgia, episodic and chronic cluster headaches, postoperative pain, neuralgias, and migraine headaches.

262. The answer is **true**.

263. The answer is **true**. Both phentolamine and clonidine are α-blockers and may be used for sympathetically mediated pain.

264. The answer is **false**. Consultants must be familiar with the legal concepts related to competency and treatment refusal and to be able to use this knowledge to diminish consultees' anxiety and to help them perform their jobs. However, though psychiatrists have often been accorded the position of legal authority by colleagues, psychiatrists do not in fact have such legal authority.

265. The answer is **c**. The failure to keep matters private is a breech of confidentiality, not a feature of malpractice proof.

266. The answer is **true**.

267. The answer is **true**.

268. The answer is **true**.

269. The answer is **false**. Physicians may terminate the treatment relationship for failure to keep appointments or for threatening behaviors or for other reasons.

270. The answer is **true**.

271. The answer is **false**. A competent adult patient has the right to refuse treatment even it is life-sustaining, and even if that decision conflicts with what a majority of others would choose under similar circumstances.

272. The answer is **false**. Such steps are considered to be euthanasia. In many states a physician who carries out such acts may be subjected to criminal prosecution.

273. The answer is **true**.

274. The answer is **false**. The court found that the state can assert its interest in preserving life and require clear and convincing evidence of a now incompetent patient's preferences in such matters before a surrogate decision maker will be allowed to refuse the treatment on the patient's behalf.

275. The answer is **false**. These facilities must inquire on admission or enrollment whether a patient has an advanced directive. If not, the patient must be offered information on the subject and an opportunity to create a directive.

276. The answer is **false**. Informed consent is required before initiation of any medical treatment, but exceptions do exist.

277. The answer is **true**.

278. The answer is **true**. The process is called therapeutic privilege.

279. The answer is **false**. It is called the materiality standard or patient-oriented standard.

280. The answer is **true**.

281. The answer is **true**.

282. The answer is **true**. The psychiatric consultant can only make a clinical assessment of the patient's capacity to function in certain areas. The court, in its determination of incompetence, usually, but not always, accepts the assessment.

283. The answer is **b**. Presence or absence of life-threatening situations is not essential to assessment of capacity.

284. The answer is **false**. The structures of the competency test vary as the risk-benefit ratio changes. In essence, there is a sliding scale for the level of competence.

285. The answer is **false**. The more favorable the risk-benefit ratio, the lower the standard for competence to consent and the higher the standard for competence to refuse.

286. The answer is **false**. One can be cognitively impaired yet still have an appreciation of risks and benefits.

287. The answer is **true**.

288. The answer is **false**. For the hospitalized infant, the key developmental challenge is to maintain the quality of attachment between parent and child.

289. The answer is **false**. The three phases of separation anxiety,

according to Bowlby, are protest, despair, and detachment.

290. The answer is **true**.

291. The answer is **true**.

292. The answer is **false**. This phase is termed detachment.

293. The answer is **true**.

294. The answer is **false**. The preschooler acts as though all life events revolve him/her. They conceptualize this phase as ego-centricity.

295. The answer is **true**. This belief system is termed body image anxiety. It leads to fear of needle sticks and surgical procedures that seem to exceed what can be explained by the painful experience alone.

296. The answer is **c**. Improper safety precautions do not form the basis for child abuse.

297. The answer is **true**.

298. The answer is **c**. Also, frequent school absences can be a sign of neglect.

299. The answer is **true**. Girls have a reported incidence of sexual abuse (38%) before the age of 18, whereas boys have a reported incidence of 15%.

300. The answer is **true**.

301. The answer is **true**. Also, the disinhibiting effects of substance abuse will increase the risk of sexual abuse.

302. The answer is **true**. Münchausen syndrome by proxy is seen when a

parent consciously distorts his/her description of the child's symptoms, or does things to the child to fabricate a picture of medical illness, and then seeks medical interventions for the child.

303. The answer is **true**.

304. The answer is **false**. Once a drug is approved for use for one condition, it may be used for another unapproved condition or by a route of administration not yet approved.

305. The answer is **false**. The typical starting dose is 18.75 to 37.5 mg qd with increments of 18.75 mg every few days thereafter until desired effects or until side effects interfere with treatment.

306. The answer is **c**. Stimulants can be safely administered to those taking antibiotics, anticonvulsants, and dermatological agents.

307. The answer is **c**. The tricyclic antidepressant imipramine is often used to treat enuresis.

308. The answer is **e**. As an α-adrenergic agent, it can be safely administered to those with asthma.

309. The answer is **c**. While hypotension can occur, bradycardia is not a common side effect of clonidine.

310. The answer is **false**. Pregnancy is not protective with respect to the emergence or persistence of psychiatric disorders.

311. The answer is **false**. Information regarding the safety of these agents is not yet available.

312. The answer is **false**. Current estimates about major cardiovascular

malformation associated with prenatal exposure to lithium are roughly 1 in 2,000.

313. The answer is **false**. The risk of developing neural tube deficits is 3% to 5%, and for spina bifida it is 1% with use of these agents.

314. The answer is **false**. Treatment of psychosis in pregnancy typically requires use of high-potency neuroleptics that have not been associated with an increased risk of congenital malformations when used in the first trimester.

315. The answer is **true**.

316. The answer is **true**.

317. The answer is **true**.

318. The answer is **a**. Advanced maternal age has not yet been associated as a risk factor for post-partum mood disorder.

319. The answer is **false**. While the signs and symptoms of postpartum depression are the same as major depression in other settings, the prevalence of postpartum depression is 10%.

320. The answer is **true**.

321. The answer is **false**. Approximately one-half of cases of liver failure in the United States are caused by alcoholic cirrhosis or alcoholic hepatitis.

322. The answer is **false**. Each center uses its own criteria for selection of organ transplant candidates and varies in their use of psychiatric risk factors or exclusionary criteria.

323. The answer is **false**. HIV infection is caused by the RNA virus HIV type 1.

324. The answer is **true**. During the process of replicating itself in the cell, the virus injures and kills the cell.

325. The answer is **true**.

326. The answer is **false**. CD-4 lymphocytes are normally greater than 800 per microliter, but the high risk for opportunistic infection occurs when the CD-4 count drops below 200 per microliter.

327. The answer is **true**. However, HIV replicates poorly in these cells producing fragments of HIV which are highly antigenic and elicit a cell-mediated immune response.

328. The answer is **d**. Other neuropsychiatric side effects of AZT are restlessness, depression, and irritability.

329. The answer is **e**. Other neuropsychiatric side effects of acyclovir are fearfulness, hyperesthesia, insomnia, and agitation.

330. The answer is **true**.

331. The answer is **false**. It is not characteristic of the AIDS dementia complex, but it is common to become delirious from some other source.

332. The answer is **true**.

333. The answer is **false**. Even demented individuals may have the capacity to make decisions and to be competent.

334. The answer is **c**. Criteria include an acquired abnormality in at least two cognitive abilities; for example,

attention, abstraction, memory, visual or spatial functions, a decline in mental status, impairment at work or activities of daily living, either acquired abnormalities in motor function or motivation, absence of clouding of consciousness, and evidence for another cause (e.g., CNS opportunistic infection) must be ruled out.

335. The answer is **false**. Trail Making Tests A and B and the Wisconsin Card Sorting Test primarily tests frontal lobe functions.

336. The answer is **false**. Psychostimulants are often useful in HIV-infected patients with poor attention and concentration.

337. The answer is **c**. Other causes of secondary mania in this population include use of AZT, D4T, steroids, ganciclovir, and procarbazine.

338. The answer is **false**. Major depressive disorder is not a normal consequence of HIV infection.

339. The answer is **false**. Peripheral neuropathy is the most common pain syndrome associated with HIV infection and affects up to 35% of patients with AIDS.

340. The answer is **true**. Zidovudine, didanosine, and D4T can each cause peripheral neuropathy.

341. The answer is **b**. Other risk factors include chronic medical illness, occupational hazards, and suicide attempts.

342. The answer is **a**. Other risk factors include risk-taking behavior, depression, and fire-setting. Burns in children and adolescents are the third leading cause of injury and death for those between the ages of 1 and 18.

343. The answer is **false**. In the first 6 months after spinal cord injury, 10% to 30% develop DSM-IV criteria for major depressive disorder.

344. The answer is **true**. Insertion of a catheter is just as likely to cause an erection as the touch of a loving hand.

345. The answer is **true**. Psychogenic erections occur in spinal cord patients who are flaccid, while reflexogenic erections occur in those who have spasticity.

346. The answer is **false**. Compassion in physicians and nurses is the most highly valued by the terminally ill.

347. The answer is **false**. Ensuring the comfort of a terminally ill person requires meticulous attention to detail, great practical knowledge, and creative ingenuity.

348. The answer is **true**. Having a gentle and appropriate sense of humor can bring relief to all parties involved in the care of the terminally ill.

349. The answer is **e**. The patient and his/her best interests is paramount, not the emotional state of their survivors.

350. The answer is **true**. Only 4% of a sample of surgical patients became emotionally upset at the time they were told about a poor prognosis.

351. The answer is **false**. The World Health Organization definition of palliative care does not mention death; it refers to the total health care of patients whose disease is not responsive to curative treatments. The goal of palliative care is the maximization of quality of life.

352. The answer is **a**. In descending order, the loss of dignity was cited by 57%, pain 46%, unworthy dying 46%, being dependent on others 33%, and tired of living 23%.

353. The answer is **true**.

354. The answer is **true**.

355. The answer is **true**.

356. The answer is **true**. In this situation, application of CPR is contrary to the standards of medical practice and is unethical.

357. The answer is **c**. General hospital psychiatric units opened in the 1930s. In 1934, 96% of psychiatric beds were under government control and generally found in state or Veteran's Administration hospitals.

358. The answer is **d**. While in certain circumstances, support of family and friends may be necessary, typically adult patients can be responsible for their own medication use.

359. The answer is **true**. There may be occasions when full informed consent may increase a patient's anxiety and make them reluctant to engage in a therapeutic medication trial, or become so suggestible that side effects may appear to develop.

360. The answer is **false**. In general, medications for the elderly should be initiated at lower doses because metabolism is often slower and excretion delayed; doses should be adjusted less frequently than in younger patients because the time required for drugs to achieve steady state levels in the elderly is often prolonged.

361. The answer is **false**. Once a drug is approved by the FDA, a physician is free to choose any approved drug for non-approved indications or by non-approved routes of administration. However, the medical record should reflect the clinical decision-making in this regard.

362. The answer is **false**. Cost effectiveness is an important concept that may reveal that an expensive drug may better prevent costly treatments and hospitalizations, and therefore be cost effective.

363. The answer is **c**. Following the synthesis of chlorpromazine in the 1950s, antipsychotics have been used widely.

364. The answer is **true**.

365. The answer is **true**. This finding probably reflects a lower affinity to D_2 dopamine receptors.

366. The answer is **true**.

367. The answer is **b**.

368. The answer is **d**.

369. The answer is **e**.

370. The answer is **a**.

371. The answer is **c**.

372. The answer is **true**. Thioridazine and mesoridazine are examples of piperidine-substituted phenothiazines that have potent anticholinergic side effects.

373. The answer is **false**. Droperidol, approved as a preanesthetic agent, is shorter-acting than is haloperidol.

374. The answer is **false**. Pimozide, a diphenylbutylpiperidine, approved for the treatment of Gilles de la Tourette's syndrome, has a half-life of several days.

375. The answer is **d**.

376. The answer is **b**.

377. The answer is **a**.

378. The answer is **c**.

379. The answer is **e**.

380. The answer is **c**.

381. The answer is **a**.

382. The answer is **e**.

383. The answer is **b**.

384. The answer is **d**.

385. The answer is **b**.

386. The answer is **b**.

387. The answer is **b**.

388. The answer is **a**.

389. The answer is **c**.

390. The answer is **a**.

391. The answer is **a**.

392. The answer is **b**.

393. The answer is **true**.

394. The answer is **true**. However, several other neuroleptics, especially haloperidol, are commonly used by the intravenous route for the treatment of agitation and delirium.

395. The answer is **true**.

396. The answer is **false**. Haloperidol decanoate has a longer half-life that allows dosing intervals of 3 to 6 weeks, whereas the half-life of fluphenazine decanoate is 7-10 days, allowing dosing every 2 weeks.

397. The answer is **false**. Blood levels of antipsychotic drugs do not correlate well with clinical response.

398. The answer is **true**.

399. The answer is **true**.

400. The answer is **true**.

401. The answer is **e**. Symptoms of Parkinson's disease tend to worsen with treatment with antipsychotics, although these agents may be necessary when psychosis complicates the illness or its treatment.

402. The answer is **e**. Typical antipsychotics may treat Huntington's disease, Tourette's syndrome, and hemiballismus, while causing torsades in higher dosages.

403. The answer is **false**. Doses are limited by the FDA to 0.3 mg per kilogram, or 20 mg per day, whichever is less.

404. The answer is **true**.

405. The answer is **true**.

406. The answer is **c**.

407. The answer is **d**.

408. The answer is **false**. 150 mg of haloperidol decanoate is approximately equivalent to 10 mg per day of oral haloperidol.

409. The answer is **false**. Clozapine has been helpful in treating L-dopa-induced psychotic symptoms.

410. The answer is **a**.

411. The answer is **false**. Greater than 95% of cases of clozapine-induced agranulocytosis occur within 6 months, with the highest risk occurring between weeks 4 and 18.

412. The answer is **false**. Most clozapine-responsive patients are effectively treated with doses of 300 to 600 mg per day in divided doses.

413. The answer is **b**. Below 600 mg per day, the risk of seizures from clozapine is 1% to 2%.

414. The answer is **d**. Clozapine causes postural hypotension, not hypertension.

415. The answer is **true**. Risperidone also has a high affinity for the D_2 dopamine receptor and the α_1 adrenergic receptor.

416. The answer is **e**. High-potency agents cause dystonia more often than do low-potency agents.

417. The answer is **e**.

418. The answer is **d**.

419. The answer is **false**. NMS is an idiosyncratic reaction to neuroleptic agents.

420. The answer is **c**. Other signs and symptoms of NMS include increased white blood cell count, increased CPK, diaphoresis, and tremor.

421. The answer is **d**. Adequate hydration is crucial as is cardiac monitoring and monitoring of inputs and outputs.

422. The answer is **true**. Dantrolene is usually given in doses of 1-3mg/kg/d for NMS.

423. The answer is **false**. At least 20% of neuroleptic-treated patients will develop tardive dyskinesia after long-term care.

424. The answer is **true**.

425. The answer is **a**. Doses greater than 800 mg per day of thioridazine are associated with increased degenerative changes with visual impairment.

426. The answer is **c**. In women, the result of hyperprolactinemia is galactorrhea or amenorrhea, or both. In men, hyperprolactinemia may cause impotence.

427. The answer is **true**.

428. The answer is **false**. Between 30% to 50% of bipolar patients develop a manic episode during treatment with an antidepressant.

429. The answer is **b**. Patients with atypical depression report hypersomnia, not insomnia. Patients with atypical depression tend to respond better to MAOIs than to TCAs.

430. The answer is **e**. Amoxapine, which possesses some neuroleptic properties, has been implicated in tardive dyskinesia.

431. The answer is **a**.

432. The answer is **d**. Typically used in doses of 150-250 mg per day, clomipramine's use is limited by its anticholinergic side effects.

433. The answer is **b**.

434. The answer is **false**. Analgesia may be achieved with levels of approximately 120 ng/ml while antidepressant levels of greater than 225 ng/ml are often required to treat depression.

435. The answer is **c**.

436. The answer is **d**.

437. The answer is **a**.

438. The answer is **b**.

439. The answer is **e**.

440. The answer is **false**. Nortriptyline's therapeutic plasma levels are 50-150 ng/ml.

441. The answer is **e**.

442. The answer is **c**.

443. The answer is **a**.

444. The answer is **b**.

445. The answer is **d**.

446. The answer is **a**.

447. The answer is **b**.

448. The answer is **c**.

449. The answer is **d**.

450. The answer is **e**.

451. The answer is **d**.

452. The answer is **a**.

453. The answer is **b**.

454. The answer is **a**.

455. The answer is **b**.

456. The answer is **c**.

457. The answer is **false**. Fluoxetine is the most potent 2D6 inhibitor of the SSRIs.

458. The answer is **true**. Fluoxetine's half-life is 2-4 days, while sertraline's half-life is 25 hours.

459. The answer is **true**.

460. The answer is **false**. L-Triiodothyronine is prescribed in doses of 25-50 mcg per day.

461. The answer is **d**. Trazodone rarely causes priapism; on occasion it is used to treat sexual dysfunction.

462. The answer is **a**.

463. The answer is **e**. Early reports found it to have antidepressant properties and MAOI activity. Its hepatotoxicity precluded iproniazid's ongoing use.

464. The answer is **true**.

465. The answer is **b**. Cade, after noting lithium's calming effect on animals, tried it on 10 manic patients and found dramatic improvement.

466. The answer is **e**. Lithium's approval for use in the United States was delayed by the deaths secondary to lithium toxicity after its unrestricted use as a salt substitute in the 1940s. In the 1950s and 1960s, its efficacy in the treatment of mania was demonstrated beyond question.

467. The answer is **c**. Lithium levels are increased by use of thiazides by 30% to 50%.

468. The answer is **true**.

469. The answer is **false**. Lithium is effective for manic episodes in approximately 70% to 80% of cases.

470. The answer is **d**.

471. The answer is **false**. No parenteral preparation of lithium is available.

472. The answer is **true**.

473. The answer is **b**. Amiloride, a potassium-sparing diuretic, markedly decreases urine volumes without a major effect on lithium or potassium serum levels as long as the patient has normal renal function.

474. The answer is **c**.

475. The answer is **b**.

476. The answer is **a**.

477. The answer is **c**. Theophylline, aminophylline, acetazolamide, caffeine, and osmotic diuretics each lower lithium levels.

478. The answer is **d**. Valproic acid is less effective in partial seizures with or without complex symptomatology.

479. The answer is **true**.

480. The answer is **true**. Peak absorption of valproic acid after oral administration occurs in 1-2 hours, while for divalproex sodium it is 3-8 hours.

481. The answer is **false**. The half-life of valproic acid is 8 hours which accounts for a t.i.d. dosing recommendation.

482. The answer is **false**. Valproic acid increases levels of GABA, the principal inhibitory neurotransmitter in the brain.

483. The answer is **c**.

484. The answer is **true**.

485. The answer is **d**.

486 The answer is **b**.

487. The answer is **d**. Phenytoin co-administration decreases carbamazepine levels, while erythromycin and INH increase levels.

488. The answer is **e**. Although each of the other syndromes mentioned are potentially fatal, they are not caused by use of carbamazepine. While 3% of carbamazepine-treated patients develop rash, Stevens-Johnson develops rarely.

489. The answer is **b**.

490. The answer is **d**. Diarrhea, insomnia, seizures, anorexia, and nausea occur with benzodiazepine withdrawal.

491. The answer is **false**. Cocaine, a highly addictive drug, does not produce a syndrome of physiological withdrawal.

492. The answer is **true**.

493. The answer is **c**.

494. The answer is **e**.

495. The answer is **a**.

496. The answer is **b**.

497. The answer is **d**.

498. The answer is **d**.

499. The answer is **c**.

500. The answer is **a**.

501. The answer is **b**.

502. The answer is **e**.

503. The answer is **b**.

504. The answer is **d**.

505. The answer is **a**.

506. The answer is **e**.

507 The answer is **c**.

508. The answer is **true**. Clorazepate has a rapid onset. Alprazolam has an intermediate onset of action.

509. The answer is **false**. Lorazepam, oxazepam, and temazepam are metabolized only by conjugation.

510. The answer is **true**.

511. The answer is **true**.

512. The answer is **true**.

513. The answer is **false**. Buspirone is a partial agonist at the $5\text{-}HT_{1A}$ receptor.

514. The answer is **true**. As a result of its extensive first-pass metabolism, only 4% of buspirone may be bioavailable.

515. The answer is **false**. Buspirone is not cross-reactive with benzodiazepines and cannot prevent benzodiazepine withdrawal symptoms.

516. The answer is **b**. Benzodiazepines prolong REM latency.

517. The answer is **true**.

518. The answer is **b**. Other agents, which compete for microsomal enzymes that increase benzodiazepine levels, are estrogen and INH.

519. The answer is **b**. The Wisconsin card sorting test helps clarify the patient's ability to maintain or shift set.

520. The answer is **false**. Psychostimulants are schedule II drugs, the most restricted class of drugs that are medically useful.

521. The answer is **true**.

522. The answer is **false**. Dextroamphetamine's half-life is 8-12 hours, while the half-life of methylphenidate is 1-2 hours.

523. The answer is **true**.

524. The answer is **true**. Chronic use of high-dose amphetamine may also produce a paranoid psychosis.

525. The answer is **d**. Narcolepsy also is associated with sleep paralysis.

526. The answer is **e**. When given in high doses, psychostimulants present with signs of adrenergic excess; including hyperactivity, increased heart rate, increased blood pressure, dry mouth, pupillary dilatation, and stereotyped behaviors.

527. The answer is **true**.

528. The answer is **true**.

529. The answer is **true**.

530. The answer is **false**. Stimulation of α-1 receptors causes vasoconstriction.

531. The answer is **true**.

532. The answer is **false**. Clonidine's principal mechanism of action appears to be as an agonist of α-2 adrenergic receptors.

533. The answer is **d**.

534. The answer is **b**. Vasodilators and β-adrenergic antagonists increase disulfiram-alcohol reactions.

535. The answer is **false**. Tacrine is a reversible inhibitor of acetylcholine esterase.

536. The answer is **true**.

537. The answer is **false**. Approximately 50% of patients on tacrine develop elevations in hepatic amino transferase activity.

538. The answer is **d**.

539. The answer is **a**.

540. The answer is **d**.

541. The answer is **a**.

542. The answer is **d**.

543. The answer is **c**.

544. The answer is **d**.

545. The answer is **e**.

546. The answer is **e**.

547. The answer is **d**.

548. The answer is **b**.

549. The answer is **d**.

550. The answer is **c**.

551. The answer is **d**.

552. The answer is **a**.

553. The answer is **e**.

554. The answer is **d**.

555. The answer is **e**.

556. The answer is **c**.

557. The answer is **c**.

558. The answer is **c**.

559. The answer is **c**.

560. The answer is **a**.

561. The answer is **c**.

562. The answer is **d**.

563. The answer is **c**.

564. The answer is **b**.

565. The answer is **b**.

566. The answer is **e**.

567. The answer is **c**.

568. The answer is **e**.

569. The answer is **c**.

570. The answer is **d**.

571. The answer is **b**.

572. The answer is **a**.

573. The answer is **a**.

574. The answer is **d**.

575. The answer is **d**.

576. The answer is **c**.

577. The answer is **c**.

578. The answer is **c**.

579. The answer is **d**.

580. The answer is **d**.

581. The answer is **d**.

582. The answer is **c**.

583. The answer is **c**.

584. The answer is **a**.

585. The answer is **a**.

586. The answer is **c**.

587. The answer is **e**.

588. The answer is **true**.

589. The answer is **true**.

590. The answer is **true**.

591. The answer is **d**.

592. The answer is **d**.

593. The answer is **e**.

594. The answer is **c**.

595. The answer is **b**.

596. The answer is **a**.

597. The answer is **d**.

598. The answer is **e**.

599. The answer is **d**.

600. The answer is **a**.

601. The answer is **c**.

602. The answer is **d**.

603. The answer is **c**.

604. The answer is **b**.

605. The answer is **b**. In general, SSRIs are not very anticholinergic, so dry mouth is infrequently associated with their usage.

606. The answer is **c**. Orthostatic hypotension is due to α_1 adrenergic receptor blockade, not muscarinic receptor blockade.

607. The answer is **d**. Blockade of the histamine H_1 receptor causes sedation, increased appetite, and weight gain.

608. The answer is **c**. Nortriptyline, doxepin, and trimipramine are tricyclic antidepressants (TCAs), while escitalopram is a selective serotonin reuptake inhibitor (SSRI).

609. The answer is **a**. The risk of seizures in bupropion-treated eating-disordered patients is higher than in bupropion-treated noneating–disordered patients.

610. The answer is **a**. Since bupropion lacks significant anticholinergic, antihistaminic, and anti-α_1 adrenergic effects, side effects (such as blurred vision, urinary retention, weight gain, sedation, and orthostatic hypotension) are relatively infrequent with its use.

611. Answer is **d**. Mirtazapine has significant histamine H_1 receptor blocking activity, which accounts for its ability to induce sedation, to increase appetite, and to cause weight gain.

612. The answer is **c**. Phenelzine and other MAOIs may interact with foods containing tyramine and with sympathomimetic drugs, leading to a lethal hypertensive crisis.

613. The answer is **a**. Relative but not absolute contraindications to the use of ECT include increased intracranial pressure, coronary artery disease, digitalis toxicity, and intracranial lesions.

614. The answer is **c**. Many patients take five to eight weeks to show significant improvement; therefore, at least six weeks of treatment with a given antidepressant is indicated. Combination of antidepressants and antianxiety drugs, to address nervousness and agitation, is relatively common in depression. Less than 60% of depressed patients typically show a robust response to treatment, with a substantial proportion of patients showing only a partial but significant improvement. Use of TCAs is commonly associated with anticholinergic side effects.

615. The answer is **c**. Those who are widowed are at greater risk for suicide than those who are divorced or married.

616. The answer is **b**. Medication may be advisable for an agitated and potentially suicidal patient who is threatening their own life or jeopardizing the safety of the staff. However, failure to cooperate, in and of itself, is not an indication for pharmacotherapy.

617. The answer is **d**. The locus coeruleus is heavily innervated by noradrenergic neurons; when it is stimulated panic may result.

618. The answer is **e**. Moreover, chest pain is common in patients with panic disorder (PD). PD occurs in 10% to 20% of patients with chest pain who present to emergency rooms. Chest pain in patients with PD results in increased usage of emergency rooms and intensive care units and accounts for an increase in cardiac work-ups.

619. The answer is **a**. Onset of symptoms after the age of 35, lack of a personal or family history of an anxiety disorder, lack of avoidance behavior, and a poor response to antipanic agents, are each factors suggestive of an organic anxiety disorder.

620. The answer is **a**. Beta-adrenergic agonists, not beta-blockers, are associated with anxiety symptoms. However, beta-blockers, have been associated with confusion and depression.

621. The answer is **c**. Diabetes (with hypoglycemic episodes), hyperthyroidism, complex partial seizures, and COPD all contribute to anxiety symptoms.

622. The answer is **b**. While GAD, PTSD, OCD, and social phobia are associated with anxiety, they are not characterized by discrete episodes which peak in intensity in 10 minutes.

623. The answer is **d**. While GAD, OCD, panic disorder, and social phobia are associated with anxiety symptoms, they do not involve exposure to a threat of death or injury.

624. The answer is **e**. Oxazepam has a slow onset of action and its half-life is 5-15 hours. Clonazepam has an intermediate onset of action and a half-life of 15-50 hours. Clorazepate has a rapid onset of action and a half-life of 30-200 hours. Lorazepam has an intermediate onset of action and a half-life of 10-20 hours. Dose equivalents are as follows: clonazepam, 0.25 mg; alprazolam, 0.5 mg; lorazepam, 1 mg; diazepam, 5 mg; clorazepate, 7.5 mg; and oxazepam, 15 mg.

625. The answer is **e**. Oxazepam, temazepam, and lorazepam require only glucuronidation by the liver; oxazepam lacks significant metabolites.

626. The answer is **c**. The half-life of the benzodiazepines listed are: alprazolam, 12-15 hours; chlordiazepoxide, 5-30 hours; clorazepate, 30-200 hours; lorazepam, 10-20 hours; and oxazepam, 5-15 hours.

627. The answer is **c**. As a rule, benzodiazepines elevate the seizure threshold. As a consequence, patients undergoing electroconvulsive therapy (ECT) generally have their benzodiazepines held prior to ECT.

628. The answer is **a**. Typically, increased gastrointestinal motility develops when withdrawing from benzodiazepines; irritability, insomnia, nervousness, and seizures may also occur.

629. The answer is **c**. Dilated pupils are typically found in response to stress or anxiety.

630. The answer is **e**. The method of payment method for psychiatric services does not in general help one's understanding of chronic stress, although it may be correlated with other indicators of social connectedness.

631. The answer is **b**. Stress responses are associated with a lowering of skin temperature.

632. The answer is **e**. Cutting down, being annoyed, feeling guilty, and having an eye-opener are four factors queried with the CAGE questionnaire. While many alcoholics believe it is easy to stop drinking, that statement is not one of the CAGE criteria.

633. The answer is **a**. Two or more positive responses on the CAGE ques-

tionnaire correlate with significant alcohol-related problems.

634. The answer is **e**. Lorazepam, because it is metabolism requires only glucuronidation, and not oxidative metabolism by the liver, is typically preferred in those with impaired hepatic function.

635. The answer is **a**. Naltrexone is an opiate antagonist.

636. The answer is **e**. Liver function needs to be monitored during disulfiram therapy because it can lead to hepatitis.

637. The answer is **e**. The prevalence of migraines is thought to be 20% in females.

638. The answer is **a**. Migraines are usually unilateral, in the frontotemporal area.

639. The answer is **b**. Cluster headaches come on quickly and peak in 5-10 minutes.

640. The answer is **d**. Propranolol is used for prophylaxis, not for acute treatment of migraine.

641. The answer is **d**. Sumatriptan is only used for acute treatment and not for the prophylaxis of migraine.

642. The answer is **d**. Restless legs syndrome is often thought of as a pre-sleep phenomenon that causes dyssomnia; it is not a parasomnia.

643. The answer is **d**. Core temperature may be recorded, but skin temperature is not.

644. The answer is **b**. Bupropion, with an amphetamine-like structure, tends to be activating, not sedating.

645. The answer is **d**. While the presence of the other conditions listed does not make one immune to snoring, obstructive sleep apnea commonly leads to loud snoring.

646. The answer is **d**. Five or more episodes of apnea or hypopnea per hour of sleep are required for the diagnosis of sleep apnea to be made.

647. The answer is **e**. Sleepwalking, a parasomnia, is not one of the diagnostic features of narcolepsy.

648. The answer is **d**.

649. The answer is **c**.

650. The answer is **b**.

651. The answer is **a**.

652. The answer is **e**.

653. The answer is **e**.

654. The answer is **a**.

655. The answer is **d**.

656. The answer is **b**.

657. The answer is **c**.

658. The answer is **b**. Actually fatigue is one of the most common complaints in ambulatory medical settings (unrelated to age), and it is more common in women than among men.

659. The answer is **e**. While anemia may cause fatigue, an isolated decrease in platelets is not associated with fatigue.

660. The answer is **true**.

661. The answer is **true**.

662. The answer is **false**. Nearly two-thirds of patients with hypochondriasis have concurrent personality disorder, and nearly three-fourths of patients with somatization disorder have concurrent personality disorder.

663. The answer is **false**. The features listed are those of hypochondriasis.

664. The answer is **false**. The features listed are those of somatization disorder.

665. The answer is **b**. Conversion disorders do not involve culturally sanctioned responses.

666. The answer is **a**. Intentionally feigned symptoms are not part of somatization disorder; they are a component of factitious disorders and malingering.

667. The answer is **c**. Denial represents a normal response to acute stress.

668. The answer is **true**.

669. The answer is **false**. Right-sided parietal lesions and sometimes subcortical lesions can cause neglect of hemiplegic limbs usually on the left side of the body.

670. The answer is **false**. Symptoms are under-reported, and patients and family members blame them on advancing age.

671. The answer is **true**.

672. The answer is **true**.

673. The answer is **d**. Shopping is an independent activity of daily living, not a basic activity of daily living.

674. The answer is **false**. Frontal lobe function is inadequately assessed by means of the MMSE.

675. The answer is **a**. Variable moods in the first few months after the diagnosis of cancer is made can be part of a normal response.

676. The answer is **e**. While the others are anti-cancer drugs they are not hormonal agents. Procarbazine and 5-fluouricil are chemotherapeutic agents, while interferon and interleukin-2 (IL-2) are biologicals.

677. The answer is **a**. Affective, behavioral, and cognitive symptoms are common with corticosteroids. As the dose of the corticosteroid increases so does the frequency of side effects.

678. The answer is **a**. Aminoglutethimide is not a dopamine blocker as are the other agents listed.

679. The answer is **d**. It is hypocalcemia, and not hypercalcemia, that is associated with tetany.

680. The answer is **d**. Although psychological reactions to the diagnosis of cancer include anxiety and depression such reactions do not result in a syndrome of delirium.

681. The answer is **c**. Paraneoplastic syndromes are associated with limbic encephalitis but not with metastatic lesions per se in the cerebrum.

682. The answer is **e**. While sumatriptan can reduce nausea and vomiting associated with migraine headaches, it is not generally used to treat post-chemotherapy nausea and vomiting.

683. The answer is **e**. Ondansetron and granisetron are both 5-HT$_3$ antagonists.

684. The answer is **c**. Metoclopramide is both a cholinergic and dopamine antagonist.

685. The answer is **b**. Palliative care is not euthanasia. The goal of palliative care is to alleviate suffering.

686. The answer is **true**.

687. The answer is **false**. The amount and detail provided to a patient should be consonant with the patient's response to general questions and with their capacity to understand and to deal with information.

688. The answer is **false**. Neuropsychiatric complications of terminal illness are often under-recognized and under-treated. Recognition may be hindered by the clinician's limited experience in diagnosing mental disorders in the setting of serious physical illness, by their difficulty in interpreting clinical information in the setting of premorbid psychiatric disorders, and by concerns about stigmatization if a diagnosis of a mental disorder is made.

689. The answer is **false**. Estimates vary, but as many as 77% of patients with terminal illness may suffer from clinically significant depression.

690. The answer is **false**. As many as 85% of all patients may develop delirium near the end of life.

691. The answer is **a**. Both dextroamphetamine and methylphenidate have a low potential for abuse in this patient population and are often the drugs of choice for depressive symptoms in patients with terminal illness.

692. The answer is **c**. When delivering bad news, it is best to be succinct. Brevity and technical simplicity are useful for communication in stressful situations.

693. The answer is **true**. Moreover, the death of a deeply loved person can cause prolonged grief. Losses are more difficult to recover from when feelings are complicated or conflicted.

694. The answer is **false**. While the loss of a pregnancy is less devastating than the death of a living child, the intensity of grief often is surprisingly severe. Physicians can help mitigate the impact of those who urge grieving parents to get over their loss quickly.

695. The answer is **d**. Most patients in this situation do not worry about the physician's theories of attribution regarding the illness.

696. The answer is **a**. In general the other feelings listed are generally more common, but there may be a circumstance where catastrophic loss is experienced, e.g., when identification with the patient and their illness is faced.

697. The answer is **true**.

698. The answer is **false**. In physician-assisted suicide, the physician provides the sufficient means of death to the patient who performs the final act. The physician who administers a lethal dose of medications to a patient with the intent to end that patient's life is performing euthanasia or committing murder.

699. The answer is **true**.

700. The answer is **true**. Competency is a legal concept. The physician in effect assesses whether the patient has capacity, and this lays the groundwork for determination of the patient's competency by a court of law.

701. The answer is **false**. The decisions of a health care proxy only come into play when the patient no longer has the capacity to make treatment decisions.

702. The answer is **true**.

703. The answer is **b**. Grief is a variable but normal response to loss.

704. The answer is **d**. Grief, in general, lasts months beyond the standard expectations or ceremonies that observe grief.

705. The answer is **e**. Pain is difficult to diagnose by use of objective tests.

706. The answer is **c**.

707. The answer is **d**.

708. The answer is **b**.

709. The answer is **a**.

710. The answer is **d**. Typically a minor injury is responsible for RSD.

711. The answer is **e**. 10 mg of parenteral methadone is equipotent to 10 mg of parenteral morphine.

712. The answer is **c**. Aprosodia may be present, but it is not a listed higher cortical function associated with dementia.

713. The answer is **b**.

714. The answer is **a**.

715. The answer is **c**.

716. The answer is **e**.

717. The answer is **d**.

718. The answer is **a**. By age 85 the prevalence of dementia may be as high as 50%.

719. The answer is **false**. Pick's disease usually affects the frontal lobes and leads to impairment in executive function and behavior.

720. The answer is **false**. Creutzfeldt-Jakob disease is a rare, rapidly progressive disorder associated with myoclonus.

721. The answer is **a**.

722. The answer is **c**.

723. The answer is **e**.

724. The answer is **d**.

725. The answer is **b**.

726. The answer is **c**.

727. The answer is **e**.

728. The answer is **a**.

729. The answer is **b**.

730. The answer is **d**.

731. The answer is **d**.

732. The answer is **e**.

733. The answer is **c**.

734. The answer is **b**.

735. The answer is **a**.

736. The answer is **e**. Visual hallucinations are common in the elderly

and in those with sensory/visual problems.

737. The answer is **false**. Many but not all complex partial seizures originate in the temporal lobe.

738. The answer is **true**.

739. The answer is **true**. The duration of a pseudo-seizure is usually more than 5 minutes.

740. The answer is **e**. The yearly incidence of brain injury following concussive syndromes secondary to closed-head injury is greater than the incidence of dementia, epilepsy, multiple sclerosis, Parkinson's disease, schizophrenia, and stroke combined.

741. The answer is **b**. Brain-injured patients are more susceptible to sedating, hypotensive, and extrapyramidal effects of neuroleptics.

742. The answer is **true**. Because CT uses ionizing radiation, it is strongly contraindicated in pregnancy.

743. The answer is **false**. T-1 images are useful for optimal visualization of normal anatomy, while T-2 weighted images detect areas of pathology.

744. The answer is **false**. MRI is better than CT for the visualization of the posterior fossa and brain stem.

745. The answer is **true**.

746. The answer is **false**. Erectile dysfunction is defined as the inability to retain or maintain a satisfying erection until completion of sexual activity causing marked distress or interpersonal difficulty. Peyronni's disease involves an erection with a curved shaft secondary to fibrosis.

747. The answer is **true**.

748. The answer is **true**.

749. The answer is **false**. There is, however, an increased risk of Ebstein's anomaly (atrialization of the right ventricle). Although the risk for congenital malformations of the heart following lithium exposure during the first trimester is 10 times that of the risk for non-lithium treated pregnant patients, the frequency of cardiac malformations is still relatively small.

750. The answer is **false**. Roughly 5% of children born to valproic-acid-treated mothers develop neural tube defects. Moreover, the risk for congenital malformations after first trimester exposure to valproic acid is 100 times that of the risk of lithium-treated pregnant women.

751. The answer is **true**. The majority of women with postpartum psychosis are eventually diagnosed as having bipolar disorder or major depression. In addition, there is a 70% to 90% risk of developing recurrent post-partum psychosis in those with a history of postpartum psychosis.

752. The answer is **true**. Lithium levels in breast-fed infants may be nearly 50% of the maternal level posing a significant risk of lithium toxicity in the infant.

753. The answer is **c**. The lifetime prevalence of bipolar disorder is 1% to 4%. However, of those with the condition only 27% are receiving medical treatment. This represents the lowest percentage of any

major psychiatric illness. Moreover, the morbidity, mortality, and disability associated with bipolar mood disorder rank above nearly all other medical disorders.

754. The answer is **b**. Other causes of secondary mania include use of steroids, anticholinergic agents, hypoglycemia, electrolyte imbalance, and stroke.

755. The answer is **d**. Liver function tests are generally not recommended because lithium rarely causes hepatitis and is not metabolized by the liver.

756. The answer is **b**. Lanugo is more typically associated with anorexia nervosa.

757. The answer is **true**. Moreover, HIV-associated dementia affects only 5% of patients with otherwise asymptomatic HIV infection. In addition, up to two-thirds of patients with AIDS-defining illness manifest HIV dementia.

758. The answer is **true**.

759. The answer is **true**.

760. The answer is **c**. Non-compliance may well be a reason to exclude a patient from a transplant list.

761. The answer is **true**. In addition, treating a celebrity enables a clinician to vicariously taste power. However, the situation that surrounds a celebrity brings out narcissistic traits in both the staff caring for the celebrity patient and in the family and staff the celebrity brings into the medical environment. The person who cares for a celebrity should ask the patient explicitly who is to be privy to information and who is not "in the loop."

762. The answer is **true**. Up to 40% of women who present with trauma have injuries secondary to battery.

763. The answer is **a**. It is an increased respiratory rate that occurs with opiate withdrawal.

764. The answer is **e**. Normal pressure hydrocephalus may be associated with ataxia, incontinence, and confusion, but it is not in general an acute life-threatening illness associated with agitation.

765. The answer is **a**. The mnemonic, WHHHIMP, helps to recall the life-threatening causes of agitation or delirium. These include Wernicke's encephalopathy, hypertension, hypoxia, hypoglycemia, intracranial bleeds, meningitis or metabolic derangement, and poisoning.

766. The answer is **b**. It is wise not to be confrontational or to promise more than you can deliver. Trust is important.

767. The answer is **false**. Safety cannot be over-emphasized. Trust your feelings when you do not feel safe with a patient and take the necessary preventive measures to manage the environment before you continue with the examination.

768. The answer is **c**. Symptoms generally develop within hours to days after initiation of steroid treatment but may arise after several months. Moreover, approximately 60% of glucocorticoid-treated patients with psychiatric symptoms are women. Even when conditions like SLE and rheumatoid arthritis, which occur more commonly in women, are excluded, the estimates of 15% to 20% of women who undergo steroid treatment develop neuropsychiatric symptoms, compared with 3% of men.

769. The answer is **false**. The vast majority of patients who develop neuropsychiatric difficulties from steroid use have no prior psychiatric illness and the presence of a psychiatric syndrome during a prior course of glucocorticoid treatment does not predict the reaction to a future course of treatment.

770. The answer is **d**. Symptoms associated with steroid withdrawal include depression, fatigue, anxiety, and confusion as well as slowed mentation, disorientation, and anorexia.

771. The answer is **e**.

772. The answer is **true**.

773. The answer is **true**.

774. The answer is **c**.

775. The answer is **a**.

776. The answer is **c**. Supplementing pyridoxine (50 to 150 mg at bedtime) may help relieve MAOI-induced pyridoxine deficiency and subsequent paresthesias.

777. The answer is **true**. In addition, TCAs often decrease the frequency of premature ventricular contractions (PVCs); however, in a minority of patients they may be proarrhythmic.

778. The answer is **false**. Lithium levels will rise with use of thiazide diuretics by roughly 25%.

779. The answer is **false**. Torsades is an alternative name for polymorphic ventricular tachycardia.

780. The answer is **true**. Moreover, they are relatively ineffective at doses below or above a specific therapeutic range.

781. The answer is **false**. These reactions are unpredictable reactions in a small number of patients and are unexpected from known pharmacokinetic and pharmacological properties.

782. The answer is **false**. While ketoconazole erythromycin, and cimetidine are inhibitors, phenytoin is an inducer.

783. The answer is **true**.

784. The answer is **true**.

785. The answer is **false**. They produce a slow decline over days to weeks.

786. The answer is **false**. The addition of an ACE inhibitor can dramatically increase lithium levels.

787. The answer is **true**.

788. The answer is **true**.

789. The answer is **true**.

790. The answer is **false**. Only a judge can declare a patient incompetent.

791. The answer is **true**.

792. The answer is **c**. While the presence of minor children may allow the treating physicians with court approval to follow a different course of action than desired by the patient, this is not something that prevents a capacity decision from being made.

793. The answer is **true**.

794. The answer is **true**.

795. The answer is **true**.

796. The answer is **true**. However, this privilege should be invoked rarely.

797. The answer is **true**.

798. The answer is **false**. Involuntary commitment in most states does not mean that the patient can be forced to accept treatment.

799. The answer is **true**.

800. The answer is **true**.